FAT, SMART AND HAPPY

FAT, SMART AND HAPPY

Find Your Weight, Lose The Guilt, and Live Stronger!

ROBERT STEWART JENNISON

L A N I A H O U S E

Owensboro, KY

Richmond, VA - Myrtle Beach, SC -

Coon Rapids, MN - Humbolt, TN - Madisonville, KY

© 2018

ISBN-13: 978-09991257-5-5 Paperback

Editor: Marla Horner Jennison

Interior Design: dream_books @ Fiverr.com

PRINTED IN THE UNITED STATES

YOU'VE BEEN WARNED. At best, this book is for information and entertainment purposes only. It was never intended to replace individualized diagnosis and treatment of health, nutrition, and fitness issues by one or more qualified medical professionals. The author and publisher disclaim any liability arising from the application of any information or opinions in this book, or from insomnia, drowsiness, or paper cuts. The mention of any individual, product or company in this book shall not be construed as an endorsement or condemnation.

I'VE BEEN HUMBLED by the remarkable depth and quality of research and writing already devoted to topics covered in *Fat, Smart and Happy*. I stand precariously on the shoulders of pioneers whose work, whether recent or published many years ago, deserves fresh exposure to a new readers. Their insight and audacity, which first appeared in dozens of books, academic journals, news articles and trade publications, has been dutifully noted at the bottom of appropriate pages. These are actual *footnotes* because the author dislikes hiding them together in the back of the book. Many other sources have been incorporated in the text, but not all were directly referenced or acknowledged, especially when the same information was available from multiple sources. All such occurrences are used with respect and gratitude and in keeping with the author's best, unlawyered understanding of Fair Use in U.S. copyright law. Any good faith comments, complaints or corrections from any source, named or unnamed, can and will be promptly addressed in subsequent printings.

I AM GRATEFUL for family and friends, especially family. My wife of 42 years, Marla Horner Jennison, has displayed superhuman strength and patience, not only with my unfiltered comments and general disregard for boundaries, but with all my career endeavors, including five long-distance relocations. As a longtime writer, reporter, editor and educator, she was fully qualified to serve as primary editor for this project. The book is thinner, smarter and happier because of her sharp eye, sharper pen, and persistence. Good job, Sugar Babe! Your check is possibly in the mail. Thanks also to sister Lee T. Jennison for sharing resources during a critical period. My mother, Elizabeth Stewart Jennison, was a math teacher at heart, but a knowledgeable writing and grammar mentor throughout my school years. My father, Dr. J.R. Jennison, was a beloved dentist and a great listener. I've been blessed by many editors who were good teachers. Special praise to the two greatest brother-owner-editors in the newspaper business, the late John and Larry Hager. I will wait to identify any others who may or may not wish to be associated with this particular sequencing of 97,000 words. Regardless, my thanks to each and every one of them.

TABLE OF CONTENTS

PART TWO // TAKING CONTROL

PART THREE // READY FOR THE WORLD

WHY WE'RE HERE

I'm not a medical doctor or professional fat person. I haven't played either one on TV. However, I have enjoyed a long career as a reporter and editor at four medium-sized daily newspapers. This book is my first opportunity to dig deep into an important national issue with enough time and resources to challenge conventional wisdom, reach my own conclusions and push the narrative in a fresh direction.

At 6 foot-1 inch, 205 pounds, I am entry-level overweight -- as opposed to underweight, "average" weight, or obese. This is according to the widely accepted but often misleading Body Mass Index (BMI) scale of intersecting heights and weights.

This book is not the work of a fat apologist or activist. I'm a journalist who decided on the topic after noticing a 50-something, exhausted and morbidly obese woman in a shopping mall just as she stopped to catch her breath and mop her brow. She will never lose that weight, I thought. But what could she realistically hope for? Painful, crumbling knees and hips? Diabetes and heart disease? More stink eye from strangers? More shaming from family? Any compassion at all? Respect? A better job? A successful marriage? A consolation prize from Oprah?

I was clueless. All I knew from a regular diet of print and television news reports was that America was in the jaws of what was being called an "obesity crisis." Certainly, we have experienced a cultural shift in eating habits. It was enabled by a hasty change in federal farm policy, then quickly profitized by corporate agribusiness and food processors. They used the best advertising available, and lots of it. Shareholders, lobbyists and their buttonholed legislators have been pocketing the residuals while two, going on three, generations of Americans have been shamed and ridiculed for cooperating with the schemers.

The obesity crisis I found during several years of research is a conspicuous absence of corporate accountability made worse by their lobbyists, complicit legislators, bare-bones regulation and a naive reliance on voluntary solutions. There are no Russians to blame, except possibly their creamy salad dressings, which are divine on salads or a Reuben sandwich.

This is serious because the Calorie Kings have managed to "externalize" their greatest cost of doing business -- the billions in additional health care spending borne by the rest of society. We haven't seen this much feigned innocence since Big Tobacco played the victim, right up to the day boxes of subpoenaed records finally confirmed decades of deception about the health risks of smoking.

Today's profiteers speak with forked tongues. It goes something like this:

- "Beloved Consumers: Instead of real and nutritious whole foods, please enjoy these addictively sweet and salty snacks and heavily processed foods which we have carefully created in our test kitchens for your pleasure and convenience."

- And then, "What happened to you? You lazy, spineless American! Why have you become fat, ill and unsightly? Regardless, we are here to help with gym memberships, fitness apps for your smartphones, and all-new, safe and effective (Wink, wink) diet plans."

You've been hearing plenty about the real and imagined health consequences of obesity. You've shouldered the blame all along by buying into the fraudulent blame claim that anyone can achieve "energy balance." You've been teased again and again with access to the "real secret" of rapid weight loss. You hear this a lot because there's money behind those messages.

What you rarely hear about (because some truths are hard to profitize) is the widespread weight-based discrimination against children and adults, especially women. They have been partially stripped of dignity and individuality by the constant repetition of false weight norms perpetuated by the fashion and entertainment industries.

Policy-makers and the health care establishment, however well-intentioned, are largely unwilling to allow a distinction between weight and fitness. And so a great, heavy, and silent majority of Americans are systematically penalized in their wages and discouraged from seeking a better education, career advancement and their rightful social status.

It's health that matters. Yet who but a handful of academics is aware of the numerous studies linking moderate "overweight" with *longer* lives? Or the hard science that confirms the dangers of cyclical weight-loss dieting? Or the hard-to-hear truth about the real impact of exercise on weight loss? And who, except for a few outspoken feminists, are talking up the benefits of loving your own fat self while eating wisely and enjoying body movement not to lose weight, but simply to feel better?

The fat acceptance movement is a long way from entering the mainstream of American consciousness. Now is your chance to be a pioneer in spreading the message that health and happiness are the perfect antidote for guilt and bias.

This certainly is not a book to promote overeating and laziness. My goal is to expose *readers of every size* to facts, opinions and new perspectives missing from most conversations about obesity-related topics, including dieting, health and discrimination. We'll try to understand why most Americans, including those who are obese, consider weight bias acceptable, even while condemning other forms of bigotry. It's all serious business, but I have tried to make this an amusing course of study. If this book came with a nutritional analysis for its content, it might look like this:

- Protein and Fiber (Facts) 80 percent of MDR.

- Fats (Opinions, anecdotes, detours) 15 percent.

- Salt and Sugars (Humor) 5 percent.

- Carbohydrates (Filler) Not a significant source!

So dig in, guilt-free, and taste it all. The early chapters cover the big picture and how we got here. Somewhere around the middle, we move to more personal topics. Start reading anywhere you want. Skip over sections that are irrelevant to you, or anything that reeks of science, whether too much or not enough. You're not likely to get lost so long as you keep the book right-side up and read each line from left to right.

I sincerely hope you enjoy and benefit from this journey to *Fat, Smart and Happy*!

Peace and love, Y'all.

Robert Stewart Jennison

July 2018

PART ONE

THE BIG, FAT ENVIRONMENT

01

FREE TO BE

Fat, Smart, and Happy! Can we agree that's a better state of mind than feeling fat, blamed and miserable? OK, then! We're all on the same page. Actually, all of these pages.

Two-thirds of Americans are a few pounds overweight, a lot overweight, or maybe even dangerously obese. Shedding that weight for more than a few months is ridiculously hard, and millions of us prove it every day.

Let's start with the elephant in the room. No, not you! You're more of a sleek and graceful gazelle. But that's beside the point. Fat has become too big a word. We're here to strip all the stigma and shame from what should be an objective reference to size. Some are more comfortable with euphemisms such as big-boned, plus-size or fluffy. Weighing in at a teensy three letters, the word fat really belongs with other, less-judgmental descriptors such as tall, thin, bald, brown-eyed or fair-skinned.

Keep that in mind as the book describes how we got fat, accepted an unhealthy share of the blame, and forgot the most basic recipes for health and happiness. When we shed the misplaced guilt, then we are free to pursue the same self-satisfaction we have believed was only available to anorexic models, gym rats, and fitness trainers to the stars.

We're not here to talk about losing weight, although there will be ample information to steer anyone safely and slowly in that direction for years to come. Primarily, we'll digest enough information about our bodies and the world around us to become more confident about ourselves and our bodies and our health. And that is huge, is it not?

Consider this book and this philosophy your lifelong, irrevocable Get Out of Guilt Free card. You're even free to snack which, I modestly suggest, is why you need your own copy of *Fat, Smart and Happy*. Leaving red wine stains or cheesy orange fingerprints on a loaner copy will always be in bad taste.

LIFE AFTER HUNGER

So let's start by tracing how two-thirds of your fellow countrymen and countrywomen came to be considered overweight.

It goes back to all the wonderful things the USA has given the world. The impressive list includes Thomas Jefferson, Thomas Edison, Henry Ford, Bill Gates, chewing gum, jazz, skyscrapers, swivel chairs, dental floss, the cotton gin and the safety pin. Equally powerful influences sprang from America's wide prairies. There, never-ending advances in agriculture science have forever freed the United States and much of the world from the scourge of food scarcity.

That's a good thing. Absolutely! Hunger is horrible -- real wasting hunger, not the inconvenient lusting for buttery bread sticks when you have to wait 20 minutes for a table at Sir Meatball. America's genius with low-cost food production also dovetailed nicely with other American inventions, including shredded wheat, the Eskimo Pie, the potato chip, the cheeseburger, charcoal briquettes, the banana split, the pop-up toaster, the self-service supermarket, and the drive-through restaurant. But there has been a massive downside to all this. Instead of hungry humans competing for a limited supply of available foods, we have transformed -- over the course of just a few generations -- to a nation of surplus food producers.

Today, the hunger games take place at the top of the food chain where multi-billion-dollar conglomerates employ the best biochemists to create inexpensive food and drinks. Most of them are rich in flavor and poor in nutrition. Next come the psychologists and packaging specialists skilled at marketing an unlimited supply of these processed products to a finite number of mouths and stomachs. The battle against hunger long won, the competition has moved on to fatter profits, a bigger share of domestic markets, and a global pursuit for new bellies to fill with cheap calories.

The resulting toxic environment now has a name: *obesogenic.*

It describes a colossal mismatch of economics and biology: newly plentiful and affordable calories versus a human genome which has survived eons of unreliable food supplies. Our tamper-proof metabolic system has not evolved or adapted.

We maintain the same genetic instructions to store and protect fat deposits. Our hormones stand guard, as always, against the possibility of famine, never getting the memo from some brain tissue about its naive attempt to restrict caloric intake or expend more energy. The body's hormonal resistance to weight loss is powerful and viral, spreading through families, communities, and nations one big butt and one pork belly at a time.

That's a challenge for anyone who has gained even a pound of fat because of a personal injury or change in medications, a shift in hormones, or a holiday season stuffed with party foods and cocktails. It's unfortunate, but weight gain is a force of nature as real as allergies and Alzheimer's and nearly as non-judgmental about picking its targets.

So there's a lot about this obesity business with deep roots in history and evolution. But above ground -- where individuals and society make constant adjustments in this little adventure called life -- the exposed limbs are bent and twisted by social, political, and economic bluster. Honk if you love capitalism, but the widest swath of devastation is caused by a glut of misinformation, junk science, and baseless blame-shifting, mostly originating with corporate spin doctors dedicated first and foremost to a fat increase in shareholder value.

SHAME AND BLAME

Discrimination based purely on weight is widely accepted as justifiable, even by many of its victims. Fat bias is perpetuated by family members, friends, teachers, coaches, physicians, Hollywood, and the news media. Fat-shaming against children is cruel and more damaging to their well-being than is the fat being demonized.

Children themselves begin to embrace fat hatred as early as age three. By age six, kids who are presented with a silhouette of an obese child respond with descriptions such as lazy, dirty, ugly, stupid, cheater and liar.

For adults -- especially women -- weight bias negatively affects relationships, education, and treatment from the medical professionals who won't look past the pounds to perform a more difficult, more useful diagnosis of a real illness. Employment discrimination in hiring, promotion, and pay is widespread and documented in several studies. It begins with resume screening and continues with performance reviews.

One study estimated that a white female 64 pounds above "average" weight was underpaid by 9 percent -- equivalent to subtracting a year and a half of education or three years of work experience. A separate study found that, according to individual weight, plus-sized white women are charged a fat tax on wages of between 5.8 percent and 24 percent. For black women, the fat tax was somewhat less, ranging from 3.3 percent to 14.6 percent.[1]

Yes, the additional costs of medical treatment for extreme obesity are also well documented. But wage offsets for fat employees are arbitrarily and unfairly distributed. According to one study by economists, the amounts deducted from pay exceed the additional costs of their health benefits.

Fat-shaming persists while deliberate weight loss rarely does.

Lose 5 or 10 percent of body weight by dieting? It's hard, but not impossible. But only a small percentage will keep it off, according to a UCLA review of 31 studies.[2] Most will regain the lost weight -- and more. Frequent dieting is, in fact, a reliable predictor of weight gain and earlier death.

Compulsive food rituals, obsessive categorization of foods as good or bad, and the exaggerated influence of fat on self-image are all symptoms of unhealthy eating disorders. Like anorexia or bulimia, dieting is an eating disorder -- and a hugely profitable industry for those who peddle exercise videos, packaged meals, dangerous or ineffective "weight-loss" supplements and all those books promising results where all else have failed.

If their plans and products actually worked more often than not, they'd eventually run out of customers. Instead, four out of five dieters will regain more weight than they lost. And when diet plans fail, guess who gets blamed?

1: Rebecca M. Puhl and Chelsea A. Heuer. Rudd Center for Food Policy & Obesity, Yale University. "The Stigma of Obesity: A Review and Update." www.obesityjournal.org. January 22, 2009.
2: "Why Diets Don't Actually Work, According to a Researcher Who Has Studied Them For Decades." Roberto A. Ferdman. *Washingtonpost.com*. May 4, 2015.

That would be you, and a bajillion other "weak-willed" dieters. Considering that weight cycling actually leads to earlier deaths, perhaps we should embrace more satisfying ways to gain weight. Cheesecake, anyone?

DELIBERATELY ADDICTIVE

Soft drinks now typically come in 20 ounce bottles sweetened with a third of a cup of sugar. (That's more sugar than I use to make a half gallon, or 64 ounces, of perfect ice tea.) Some of the most popular children's cereals are more than half sugar by weight. Their makers are pleased to tell us they are merely offering choices to consumers, and healthy ones at that.

Honey is one of the three sweeteners in its first four ingredients of a popular brand. It's 56 percent sugar, yet the Mom-assuring message on the box is "Good Source of Vitamin D." Ditto for packaging for an equally sweet powdered oat concoction with ersatz marshmallows. One such store brand is 48 percent sugar by weight, yet it claims to be is an "excellent source" of iron and Vitamin C. Why, we'd be fools not to eat them. And we couldn't stop if we tried. They are among thousands of foods heavily processed with added salt, fats and sugar, each painstakingly designed and tested to be simply irresistible, yet not so satisfying that we will know when we've had enough. "Betcha can't eat just one?" That's not a wager. That's a promise.

Salts, sugars, and fats are the pillars of food processing. Our tongues love the taste and texture, but that's just the teaser. Studies with animals and humans have shown that fats and sugars alter brain responses in ways that closely resemble addiction to drugs. Other studies have shown how rich, sweet foods cause the brain to release pleasure-inducing opiates similar to the high from narcotics. So it's not surprising that the same meds prescribed to reduce an addict's brain response to opiates also make sweets less appealing.

Comparing soft drinks and snack foods to addictive, illicit drugs is unfair, I agree. And here is why: Neighborhood drug dealers don't get to advertise on the internet, television, buses, billboards, and high school scoreboards.

KIDSTUFF

To get their message to children and adolescents without drawing too much pushback from parents and regulators, the carbs-and-calorie industries have used many of the techniques practiced a generation earlier by tobacco companies.

Instead of handsome cowboys and cartoon Joe Camel, the likable salesmen are characters from popular children's cartoons. Frequent promotional ties to blockbuster movies keep the advertising fresh and relatable. Thus far, Big Food has succeeded in forestalling any tough regulation or punitive taxes the same way Big Tobacco did for many years: the industry just continues to deny there is a problem while offering to take the lead in attacking the non-problem through self-regulation.

But despite the fast-food industry's promise a decade ago to use more discretion, children's exposure to TV ads increased by a third over one six-year comparison. Burger King and McDonald's pledged to promote healthier menu choices to children. Instead, the marketing emphasis switched to toy giveaways and kid-centric websites such as HappyMeal.com to build brand loyalty.[3]

With fast food companies spending more than $4 billion on advertising, you can be sure the ads are carefully constructed and placed. Hispanic-American preschoolers see about 300 Spanish-language food commercials each year. McDonald's and KFC have successfully targeted African-American youth with TV advertisements, websites and online advertising. Nationwide, black teens see 75 percent more ads for KFC and McDonald's than do white teens.

The industry is happy to describe its approach as marketing that is responsive to changing demographics and customer demand. The industry would not call it racial profiling.

STEALTH BOMBERS

Hiding behind the industry's unavoidable paid advertising are equally powerful stealth campaigns to co-opt opinion leaders and policy makers. In the same way drug companies have managed to influence the scientific record to

---

3: "Fast Food FACTS 2013." *Rudd Center for Food Policy & Obesity.*

make their products appear safer and more effective, food and beverage makers have stood modestly in the shadows while spending millions to underwrite their versions of nutritional research.

A review of about 200 published scientific papers on the health effects of milk, soft drinks and fruit juices found only a fourth had no corporate sponsorship at all. Is it any wonder that industry-funded studies are four times more likely to report favorable outcomes than independently funded research?

There are countless other examples at the local, state, national and global level where the giants of food and drink have covertly undermined the efforts of opposition groups, health agencies and lawmakers. When an arm of the World Health Organization became too cash-strapped to continue its rejection of industry funding, Coca-Cola, Nestle and Unilever stepped up with $350,000 to fight diseases associated with unhealthy diets in Mexico. That nation has the honor of the highest per capita soft drink consumption in the world -- 45 gallons a year. That's 38 percent more sugar and bubbles than Americans drink (an immodest 31 gallons per year).[4]

Could a sugar tax on soft drinks -- even one with revenue earmarked for athletic and nutrition programs -- ever succeed in containing or reversing the obesogenic environment? Soft drink makers seem to think so, as evidenced by their extensive and expensive push-back campaigns. In Richmond, California, a retired cardiologist and city council member tried to win support for a one-cent-per-ounce tax. He campaigned by pulling a little red wagon loaded with 40 pounds of loose sugar. The sparkling, white mound graphically represented the annual sweetener consumption of *each child* in the community.

Supporters of the tax referendum raised $30,000 for a heartfelt mail campaign. Meanwhile, a local "grassroots" organization formed to oppose the tax got some input from the American Beverage Association. The free advice came with more than $2 million for paid advertising. The Forces of Sugar repeatedly told voters the tax would be a burden for small businesses and "hit the poor and working people the hardest." Well, so does obesity, but the soda tax was tarred, feathered and voted down.

4: Duff Wilson and Adam Kerlin. "Special Report: Food, Beverage Industry Pays For Seat At Health-Policy Table." *Reuters.com*. October 19, 2012.

Blacks and Hispanics also have disproportionately higher rates of obesity, diabetes, and heart disease. So why did the NAACP and Hispanic Federation each file legal briefs to oppose former New York City Mayor Michael Bloomberg's effort to merely downsize soda servings in restaurants? Maybe they were really thirsty. For certain, the two groups had received sponsorships and contributions totaling $200,000 and pocket change from Pepsi and Coca-Cola in the previous two years. Oh, and the law firm preparing court documents on their behalf was Coke's go-to law legal team in Atlanta.

When your products are being linked to hugely expensive health concerns, you donate soft drinks to a hospital employee picnic. Or send a check. In recent years, Coke and Pepsi have given millions of dollars to be official sponsors or partners with the American Academy of Pediatrics, the American Cancer Society, the American College of Cardiology, the American College of Sports Medicine and the Congressional Hispanic Caucus Institute. Big Soda's tone-deaf, philanthro-marketing Hall of Fame would include Coke's $125,000 gift to the American Diabetes Association and a $1 million donation to the American Academy of Pediatric Dentistry.

Your local nutrition professionals are understandably embarrassed because their 73,000-member national umbrella group each year welcomes foxes into their hen house. Specifically, the Academy of Nutrition and Dietetics routinely partners with Coca-Cola, PepsiCo, Mars, Hershey and Nestle. At one of the academy's national conferences, Nestle paid $50,000 to host a two-hour "nutrition symposium" about "optimal hydration." Many of the 10,000 registered dietitians attending earned continuing education credits by boarding a bus for a full-day field trip to the -- I am not making this up -- Hershey Center for Health and Nutrition.

The dietitians' trade association is active politically in matters affecting its members, but when the food and drink giants mobilize to oppose sugar taxes or labeling for trans-fats or genetically modified foods, the nutritionist group lies low or sides with industry.

All that six- and seven-digit lubrication sounds like big money to most of us, but it is penny poker compared to when Congress or state legislatures dare to consider soda taxes or any kind of regulation. When New York's governor proposed a penny-per-ounce soda tax and excise taxes on syrups in 2010, drink makers spent $12.8 million on direct lobbying expenses and millions more on paid advertising. PepsiCo threatened to relocate its New York headquarters and 1,000 jobs.

The measures died. Pepsi got a $4 million economic development grant to stick around. Refreshments were served. Forgiveness reigned.

As for our do-nothing Congress, be assured that doing nothing is an industry unto itself. In 2005, the soda industry spent nearly $1.3 million twisting arms on Capitol Hill. By 2009, when a Senate Finance Committee was considering a national sugar tax, the soft drink makers upped their declared lobbying expenses by a factor of 31 to more than $40 million. By 2010, with the threat of new federal taxes long since buried, the industry kept up the pressure with a $22 million lobbying effort.

THE CRUMBLING PYRAMID

Even the saintly Food Pyramid -- perhaps the most widely known graphic in the United States -- has been regularly revised to reflect the bruising negotiations between nutritionists and food producers. The U.S. Department of Agriculture's "Basic Four" food guide premiered in 1958 with its recommendations for minimum daily servings of each food group to prevent nutritional deficiencies. That evolved into the Food Pyramid every student and parent recognized as rock-solid advice. At its foundation, it said to eat up to 11 servings daily of breads, rice and pasta, along with two to five servings each of fruits and vegetables, and two or three servings of protein-rich foods including meats and dairy. The small triangle at the top represented fats and added sugars, which were to be "used sparingly."

Food producers were happy with the "Eat More" message in the days when nutrition problems were linked to hunger. But rising obesity rates in the 1990s turned the fine print of the Pyramid's recommendations from representing minimum servings per day to maximums. The new "Eat Less" emphasis did not resonate with producers. They responded forcefully through their powerful trade associations.

The House Appropriations Committee capitulated by diminishing the administrative influence of what was then called the Department of Health and

Human Services. It assigned lead agency status for dietary guidance to the more producer-friendly Department of Agriculture. In 2005, after a year of hearings and debate, the hierarchy of the original pyramid was replaced with one that appeared to give equal value to all food groups, and added a stick figure climbing stairs to represent industry's emphasis on "energy balance." The accompanying dietary guidelines were nutritionally sound and available online, but the new MyPyramid graphic was clearly designed to be unclear about what foods to eat less of.

Five years later, there was an influential, tall and toned parent of two daughters living in Washington, and her husband was President of the United States. The official dietary guidelines were due for revision again in 2010 and, for the first time, the advisory committee felt empowered to state the obvious: A majority of Americans were (and still are) overweight or obese, yet undernourished as measured by several key nutrients. They eat too few vegetables and whole grains, and too much added sugar, solid fats, refined grains and salt.

The 2010 guidelines also came with a meaningful replacement for the MyPyramid graphic. Hearkening back to the wholesome days of the basic four food groups, the new MyPlate devoted its two largest servings to vegetables and mostly whole grains, depicted a slightly smaller space for fruits and protein and a cup-size portion on the side for dairy. The new icon is blissfully free of fat, added sugar and politics. Score one for former First Lady Michelle Obama and other advocates of sound nutrition.

But have you ever seen it? Perhaps once on the evening news or in a newspaper within 24 hours of its unveiling. Since then, however, you and your children have subsequently seen thousands of billboards, television ads and internet mentions for all the processed foods and drinks blacklisted by the nutritionists who fought to make MyPlate meaningful. The budget to promote healthy foods is minuscule. One study found that for each healthy message a teenager sees, he or she is exposed to 127 pitches for manufactured foods high in sugar, salt and/or fats. We're talking about 6,000 unhealthy ad impressions per teen per year. The only way nutrition advocates could make an equally strong impression promoting healthy foods on a tiny budget would be to release a NSFW graphic with a masculine arrangement of a banana and two lemons.

KIDS COUNT

Most of today's adults will live out their lifetimes with some accumulated fat. But what about the children? Not so long ago, their pudgy cheeks were considered cute and ripe for a loving pinch. Now, chubby is shorthand for Slurpees and sloth. The yearly increases in the percentage of overweight kids has finally reached a plateau, but the numbers still warrant monitoring, especially among blacks and Latinos, which are disproportionately high compared to whites.

Rather than using BMI data, overweight and obesity tags for children are based on the range of weight for all kids in the same age group. The 10 percent of peers within the 85th to 95th percentile by weight are classified as overweight; those above the 95th percentile (the heaviest 5 percent) get the obese label.

According to data compiled through 2014 by the U.S. Centers for Disease Control[5]:

A third of all children (age 2 to 19) are overweight (16.2 percent) or obese (17.2 percent). Differences by gender have narrowed to half a percentage point.

At 17.2 percent, the number of obese children has tripled since 1980 (5.5 percent). However, attention to this highest-risk group has begun to pay dividends. For the past decade, obesity rates for children have been stable -- even declining in some years.

But children have gotten heavier earlier in life, and they keep gaining. In the age 2 to 5 group, 8.9 percent are obese; ages 6 to 11, 17.5 percent; and ages 12 to 19, 20.5 percent. Racial and ethnic differences also are prominent. The obesity rate for Asian kids is 8.6 percent; whites, 14.7 percent; blacks, 19.5 percent; and Latino, 21.9 percent.

What about the schools? Schools have the gymnasiums, athletic fields and cafeterias. Where better to institutionalize the good eating habits that are being marginalized everywhere else? Schools are making a difference, but healthy meals start with the leafy green of money. The last few years have mainly focused on undoing the damage to the last few decades, beginning in the 1970s

---

5: Cheryl D. Fryar, M.S.P.H., and others. "Prevalence of Overweight and Obesity Among Children and Adolescents Aged 2–19 Years: United States, 1963–1965 Through 2013–2014." *U.S. Centers for Disease Control and Prevention, National Center for Health Statistics.*

with the decade's shifting emphasis toward technology and creating a world-class workforce.

The federal mandate called Title IX required gender equity throughout the curriculum, including athletics. To offset that added expense, many high schools responded with the gender-neutral tack of eliminating some physical education classes completely. Today, many school districts are still replacing actual P. E .classes with *online* options. I poo you not.

And local school boards can't seem to wean themselves from negotiating lucrative contracts for "pouring rights." Pepsi and Coke often compete head-to-head for an exclusive presence in schools that often includes soda machines in school hallways and advertising space on football scoreboards. With a standard markup of $1 on a 20-ounce bottle of pop, a school district with 10,000 students can easily net a sweet $25,000 each week.

An independent study of state funding of school food services found a wide range of efforts and graded them from A to F, but the geography and politics of those states were such a hodgepodge as to defy stereotypes, let alone identify a successful blueprint for other states to follow. That leaves Congress to step up or step back. It has done both. In 2010, the Healthy, Hunger-Free Kids Act sailed through the House and Senate and gave the USDA authority to set higher nutrition standards for the $14 billion school lunch and breakfast programs. The guidelines, approved in 2012, discouraged highly-processed foods produced in commercial kitchens and promoted real cooking of real foods with more fruits, vegetables and whole grains.

By the spring of 2014, 90 percent of schools districts were in compliance. Even so, the nation's school cafeteria directors, as represented by the School Nutrition Association, began directly lobbying Congress for exceptions and delays, citing increased costs and tons of wasted foods. Perhaps there were other motivating factors. Half of their association's $10 million operating budget comes from the food industry, including the makers of snack foods and pizza that were now competing with local growers of fruits and vegetables.

Teaching children raised on sweet and salty foods to embrace whole foods will be a long slog. In fact, one of the most successful food-related programs in New York City is one that is saving the city up to $50 per ton on landfill costs by composting the half-eaten apples, bananas and other nutritious garbage harvested from lunchroom trays. "We expected these challenges, particularly among our oldest kids, who've grown up eating junk food," said then-First Lady Michelle Obama, who had made solutions to childhood obesity her top priority. "But what we did not expect was for the grown-ups to . . . go along with them and say 'Well, this is too hard, it costs too much money. So let's just stop.'"

ADULT CONTENT

So we're all in a tizzy about how to address a public health issue that is defined by a rather arbitrary and misleading system of measurement. Red Flag No. 1: the methodology behind the Body Mass Index scale dates back to the 1850s and crude, even racist, efforts to equate human averages with normalcy and to link abnormal physical attributes to antisocial behaviors. The mathematical formula of weight divided by height (squared!) was intended to mask individual differences in a population and still produce a meaningful numeric shorthand for health.

Like a teacher's grade on an essay, a credit score, or the official report of an officer-involved shooting, BMI tells a story. But not the whole story.

Regardless, here's the currently accepted standard for adults age 20 and over:

- Normal weight, BMI 18.5 to 25

- Overweight, BMI 25 to 30

- Moderately Obese, BMI 30 to 35

- Severely obese, BMI 35 to 40

- Extremely (also called very severely) obese, BMI 40 and up

The widely accepted definition for "morbidly obese" is even more inclusive. A man or woman fits that category with a BMI of 40 or more, a body weight 100 pounds above "ideal weight," or by having BMI above 35 while experiencing obesity-related health conditions, such as high blood pressure or diabetes.

With more than two-thirds of all adults in the U.S. now being counted as above "normal" weight, federal agencies and private foundations which track the trends in the U.S. have all but ignored the "merely overweight" category in their reports and outreach. Now the focus is on the increasing numbers of men and women in the obese subcategories. Here is why:

Nationally, nearly 38 percent of adults are obese. [6]

Nearly 8 percent are extremely obese.

Obesity rates are higher among women (40.4 percent) compared to men (35.0 percent). Women are also almost twice as likely (9.9 percent) to be extremely obese compared to men (5.5 percent).

There are significant racial and ethnic inequities. Obesity rates are higher among blacks (48.4 percent) and Latinos (42.6 percent) than among whites (36.4 percent) and Asian Americans (12.6 percent).

The inequities are highest among women: blacks have an obesity rate of 57.2 percent, Latinos of 46.9 percent, whites of 38.2 percent and Asians of 12.4 percent. For men, Latinos have a rate of 37.9 percent, blacks of 38.0 percent and whites of 34.7 percent. And black women (16.8 percent) are more likely to be extremely obese than white women (9.7 percent).

WEIGHING IN

Of course, it took some significant increases over four decades for obesity to earn the "crisis" designation now paired with the word as routinely as Oreos + milk. Since the early 1960s, the prevalence of obesity more than doubled, increasing from 13.4 percent to 38.2 percent among U.S. adults. The biggest surge in belt sizes occurred between the mid-1970s to the mid-1990s. Since then, however, the nation's weight curve for the gently overweight has flattened out. It's the steady increase in hardcore obesity that will guarantee a continued demand for jeans and sweats with two or more X's in the sizing.

In the unabridged timeline of civilization, the phenomenon of surplus calories is but a few grains of sand through the hourglass. Imagine the abrupt

---

6: K.M Flegal and others. "Trends in Obesity Among Adults in the United States, 2005 to 2014." *JAMA.* 2016.

onset of stretch marks and obesity if the earliest hunter-gatherers were suddenly presented with 24/7 access to soft drinks, fast food and modern supermarkets. The newly fattened would not be ashamed or hiding in caves. They would be struttin' their stuff, according to Steven Shapin, a Harvard professor and science historian. Throughout most of history, physical heft was seen as a visible mark of power, affluence, and even good humor. So it's hard to avoid the conclusion, Shapin says, that labeling someone as fat *didn't become derogatory until even the poor could afford surplus calories.*[7]

Such prejudices are clearly societal and easily passed from person to person and generation to generation. In fact, prejudices against thinness are still the norm in many parts of the world, particularly in regions that Westerners arrogantly dismiss as uncivilized.

Witness this scene at a health clinic in Saharan Niger. Sociologist Rebecca Popenoe, who spent four years living among the desert Arabs, was amused to watch visiting Nigerian nurses take their turns climbing on the scales to be weighed. "Unlike women in the West, however, who learn at an early age to remove shoes and as much clothing as possible before stepping on the scale for its verdict, the Nigerian nurses all put clothes *on*. They nonchalantly picked up shawls, sweaters, and any other loose items of clothing they had with them before stepping on the scale," she observed. "Taking their shoes off to weigh themselves was out of the question, because this would subvert their goal, which was to weigh as much as possible." [8]

The Westerner learned that even though the men of the villages were admired for being active and slender, girls learned at an early age they are expected to eat oversized portions of grains and milk in order to achieve the heft that is considered both sexy and ideal as they prepare for marriage. Stretch marks are romanticized in song. It's not impressive enough to get stretch marks on their stomachs, the women explained to the uncomfortably thin American. The real achievement, they shared, is earning stretch marks on the arms and legs.[9]

The world is still dotted with cultures, chiefly African, Arabic, Indian and

7: "Eat and Run: Why We're So Fat," Steven Shapin, Jan. 16, 2006, *The New Yorker.*
8: "Ideal," © 2004 by Rebecca Popenoe, one of a collection of essays in *Fat: The Anthology of an Obsession*, Jeremy P. Tarcher / Penguin, New York.
9: Ditto.

Pacific Islander, where collar bones and trim tummies are seen as unattractive. It is only the influence of Westerners that has turned those happy self-images of beauty and health to worrisome self-loathing.

TIME FOR A TRUCE

In the U.S., the negative stigma is sufficient to sustain what one economist has called a multi-billion Obesity Industry. William L. Weiss, a professor of management at Seattle University, counted not only the groups which help create the weight gain — chiefly the fast food and soft drink industries — but also the sectors which directly profit from the resulting weight gains and efforts to take it off. Again we're talking billions-with-a-B: $9.3 billion in annual revenues for liposuction and weight-loss surgeries, $5.29 billion for medically supervised diet programs and commercial weight loss centers, and $22.5 billion for health clubs. Weiss, who has been critical of profiteers on both ends of the Obesity Industry, added another $157 billion to represent the cost of medical treatments for obesity-related diseases. It adds up to a plus-size industry with total revenues of perhaps $400 billion.[10]

Weiss believes the beneficiaries of the fat economy are only outwardly interested in finding real cures and promoting lasting change. The natural forces of capitalism are fully at play, he says, "and both industries -- those selling junk food and those selling fat cures -- depend for their future on a prevalence of obesity." [11]

J. Eric Oliver, a University of Chicago political scientist, agrees that obesity has reached the level of discord typical of controversies which split policy-makers and pundits. "If you're on the political right, obesity is indicative of moral failure. If you are on the left, it means rampaging global capitalism."[12]

William Saletan, a columnist for the Slate website, was particularly impressed with a British study of 5,000 pairs of identical or fraternal twins which concluded that 77 percent of the factors determining thinness or fatness

---

10: "When the Interests of Industry are in Conflict with the Public Health: The Case of Obesity," William L. Weiss, *Journal of Health Care Management*. 2005. (These numbers, originally published in 2004, have been adjusted here for inflation to 2014. Actual amounts, however, are probably much larger because of real growth factors.)
11: Ditto.
12: Gina Kolata. "Study Aside, Fat-Fighting Industry Continues Mission." *New York Times,* April 29, 2005.

are genetic and hereditary. Self-identified as someone who eats like a horse without gaining weight, he says "Those of us who don't get fat should stifle our piety. We need to think of obesity the way we think of alcoholism or allergies: as an unevenly distributed biological predisposition to seek or suffer harm from common environmental factors. Yes, we should struggle against it," he says. "But it's more of a struggle for some than others." [13]

Agreed. And simply by acknowledging the powerful influence of the obesogenic environment and accepting our hardwired history of girding for famine, we are liberated to pursue new cultural, medical, and political priorities. So! Let us share three cheers and a beer for the end of fat-shaming. Welcome the era of acceptance, tolerance, and unbiased health goals for everyone, regardless of size.

13: William Saletan. "Obesity Genetics and Responsibility." www.slate.com. February 15, 2008.

02

ROUNDNESS, SQUARED

Conventional wisdom holds that a person's weight is a fair and reliable measure of that person's health. It even qualifies as common sense to anyone who believes that a person's character is revealed by his or her height, bank account or skin color.

So . . . When someone is judged to be fat *and* healthy, is that an "obesity paradox," as it's often described, or just a meaningless contradiction in the tradition of "open secret," "original copy," "jumbo shrimp" or "honest politician?"

To be sure, heavy-but-healthy doesn't match the official thinking of the American Medical Association. In 2013, the 225,000-member AMA reacted to America's growing "obesity crisis" by officially agreeing to classify obesity itself as a disease. Proponents said obesity meets the definition of disease as a condition that impairs some aspect of normal functioning, may be caused by genetic factors (true), and decreases life expectancy (except, "paradoxically," when the opposite is true!).

Cooler heads argued in vain that obesity is not a disease but a side effect resulting from a thyroid imbalance, arthritis, insulin resistance, depression, prescribed medications, sleep apnea, smoking cessation, injuries or dieting. And there's a paradox right there: dieting itself meets all the criteria experts use to classify an eating disorder.

The AMA's move to legitimize obesity itself as a disease was welcome news to the billion-dollar pharmaceutical industry which has already reaped billions in profits by targeting such public health scourges as social anxiety, occasional heartburn and toenail fungus. We have to be happy for that one shy guy somewhere who is wearing flip-flops and reluctantly entering a crowded chili parlor.

The obesity-as-disease determination is already putting pressure on the Food and Drug Administration to approve doubtable new weight-loss drugs and procedures, and for insurance companies to cover the expense. Family physicians, in turn, will have additional cover when prematurely diagnosing patients on the basis of their weight alone, rather than a personalized assessment of genetic history, body type, diet and exercise habits.

I get it. Obesity has long been *associated with* certain maladies -- most convincingly with hip and knee joints buckled by years of bearing excessive weight. But associations are too often misrepresented as cause → effect. There is, for example, strong science that shows diabetes can contribute to weight gain, not just the other way around.

WHEN BMI LIES

You know the moth-eaten maxim: Being overweight ups the risk for heart disease, diabetes and an untimely death. But a massive review of 97 different studies with a combined sample of more than 2.8 million men and women again confirmed that while the *upper extremes* of obesity can shorten life, being overweight (BMI 25-30) or moderately obese (BMI 30-35) *does not shorten life*. In fact, the overweight can look forward to more years with the grandchildren than those classified in the "normal" BMI range 18.5 – 25.[14]

The study was equally clear in concluding that the increased rate of death for the severely and morbidly obese (BMI 35 and up and up) was a suitably morbid 29 percent. Now, you might reasonably be thinking a study like this -- so inhospitable to the conventional wisdom about fat -- was probably paid for by something like The Foundation for Fudge, Fondue and French Fries. And I would admire your skepticism. We're going to get along just fine. But this research, published by the Journal of the Medical Association Network,

---

14: Katherine M. Flegal and others. "Association of All-Cause Mortality With Overweight and Obesity Using Standard Body Mass Index Categories." Journal of the American Medical Association. January 2, 2013.

was conducted by the U.S. Centers for Disease Control and Prevention and the National Cancer Institute -- with no external funding.[15] In my research notes, I always pencil in a dollar sign next to any suspicious studies and sources. Instead, this one got a big ole smiley face.

The researchers said that their findings were consistent with other observations of lower mortality among overweight and moderately obese patients. Doctors have also observed in practice that heavy patients with kidney or heart failure often fare better than thinner patients. That's partly because body fat can have an anti-inflammatory effect on the cardiovascular system,[16] and that's a good thing.

"It might simply be that chronic illness is a metabolically demanding state, and people who are overweight have greater metabolic reserves to deal with the demand," said an editorial accompanying one study.[17]

Dr. David Katz, director of a prevention research center at Yale University, said the CDC study is clear that the upper extremes of obesity are not a healthy place to be. "Your weight is a moving target, and usually in the wrong direction," said Katz, who was not part of the research team. "This study suggests that if the basis for defining 'overweight' is adverse health effects, we may want to raise the threshold. The definition of 'overweight' should begin where health risks begin."[18]

Paul Campos, a long-time critic of obesity hysteria, said the CDC finding should surprise only those who assume the public health definition of normal or healthy weight "is actually supported by the medical literature."[19] Campos is a professor of law at the University of Colorado, Boulder who made his case in a 2004 book, *The Obesity Myth: Why America's Obsession with Weight is Hazardous to Your Health.*

In his reaction to the CDC study published in the New York Times, Campos again ridiculed a system of diagnosis by benchmarks. "Baselessly

---

15: Ditto.
16: Claire E. Hastie and others. "Obesity Paradox in a Cohort of 4,880 Consecutive Patients Undergoing Percutaneous Coronary Intervention." European Heart Journal. 2010.
17: Wolfram Doehner and others. "The Obesity Paradox: Weighing the Benefit." European Heart Journal. 2010.
18: Dan Childs. "Is Being Overweight Really Bad for You? abcnews.go.com. January 1, 2013.
19: Paul Campos. "Our Absurd Fear of Fat." The New York Times. January 2, 2013.

categorizing at least 130 million Americans . . . as people in need of 'treatment' for their 'condition' serves the economic interest of, among others, the multibillion-dollar weight industry and large pharmaceutical companies, which have invested a great deal of money in winning the goodwill of those who will determine the regulatory fate of the next generation of diet drugs."[20]

Assigning an individual to a weight category defined by his or her weight alone is a powerful reinforcement of negative stereotypes and prejudices. Weight benchmarks and branding are distractions, at best, and dangerous -- even lethal -- when they interfere with individualized medical diagnosis and treatment. To whatever extent modern medicine relies on a formula as crudely calculated and widely misinterpreted as BMI, public health takes the hit.

PENNY SCALES AND FAIRY TALES

The widespread effort to put an exact figure on a human's weight began as a novelty and gimmick. In the U.S. during the mid-1800s, manufacturers of heavy scales built to weigh wagon loads of farm produce began to tout their accuracy by measuring the weight of entire families which lined up for the honor at county fairs. By the 1930s there would be a half million individual sized "penny scales" spread throughout the country, first locating in the high-traffic areas such as railway stations, subways, and pharmacies, then dime stores, banks and office buildings.[21]

Soon, scale manufacturers and magazine publishers were willing and able to promulgate fat-phobia as a means of equating weight with beauty, health, and happiness. Yet their influence was small potatoes compared to the harvest of hysteria sewn by actuaries and reaped by America's burgeoning life insurance industry.

Millions of Americans -- first the middle class and then the working poor -- were being sold on the importance of planning for their funerals and buying private life insurance. By 1924, some 92 million policies worth $2.2 billion were in place. Life insurance was big business and responsible for many of the first skyscrapers to rise in America's cities. [22]

20: Ditto.
21: Hillel Schwartz. *Never Satisfied: A Cultural History of Diets, Fantasies & Fat. Anchor Books*. Double-
    day. New York. 1986. First Anchor Books edition, 1990.
22: Schwartz.

Naturally, stockholder-owned insurance companies attempted to minimize their risk exposure by screening policy applicants, always looking for something besides age and occupation that would predict a "premature" death. ("On the Bomb Squad, you say? Lemme just make a note of that.") Height and weight information was easy and inexpensive to collect from each new policy applicant, readily compiled in a massive database, and continuously updated with the age at which each policyholder died. Beginning with its first appearance in 1897, the insurance industry's height-weight tables were widely accepted as a useful yardstick -- a subjective, scientific predictor of mortality.[23]

The earliest tables were sensible to the extent that the data was broken down not only by gender, but also age group. The consensus in the early 1900s was that weight was not a factor in mortality unless someone was at least 20 percent above the "average" weight. True or not, policyholders in that category were routinely charged higher premiums, even though many doctors at the time argued than thin people were more vulnerable to diseases of the day, especially tuberculosis and pneumonia. As subsequent studies and revisions would confirm, the charts were based on unreliable data and then skewed to support erroneous assumptions. "Tables of 'ideal' or 'desirable' weight make about as much sense as tables of ideal or desirable heights," as Glenn Gaesser wrote in *Big Fat Lies*.[24]

To start with, policyholders generally reported their own weights and did so only once -- when they first purchased a policy. Gaesser found a bigger weakness when he compared the touted height-weight charts to the raw data on which there were reputedly based -- data he says actually correlated "overweight" with *improved* mortality for some age and gender groups. Nevertheless, the public impact of the charts spread like influenza, especially in 1942 when the Metropolitan Life Insurance Company managed to create a national obesity epidemic overnight. When it published new weight tables, the descriptive term "average" weight had been replaced with "ideal" weight. And now there was no consideration for normal, gradual weight gain over many years. The "ideal" weight for those aged 20-29 was now the target weight for *all* age groups.

23: Gaesser, Glenn A., Ph.D. *Big Fat Lies*. New York: Fawcett Columbine, 1996. This section on height-weight tables draws heavily on Gaesser's work. Gaesser is currently a professor of exercise science and health at Arizona State University. His entire book is highly recommended reading for professionals and laymen.
24: Gaesser.

The fashion and fitness industries kept weight worries on the front burners in the 1960s and 1970s. Ironically it was MetLife, in 1983, which attempted to rein in the frenzy. It had good reason. The most recent actuarial data, released in 1979, dared to report that the optimum weights for longevity had increased by as much as 17 percent compared to its findings a generation earlier. MetLife still made no allowances for age, but generously upped overall targets. That 5-foot-4 woman of "medium" frame who was expected to weigh 113-126 pound in 1959 was, in 1983, permitted to tip the scales at up to 138 pounds.[25] Heck, MetLife even admitted its recommended weights would not minimize illness and disease, even saying the company did not use its own charts in computing premiums.[26]

You may assume, quite correctly, this softer approach from insurers did not sit well with the massive public and private organizations which depended in part on defining obesity itself as a "killer disease" in order to raise and spend millions of dollars.

BMI: ROUNDNESS, SQUARED

What fat-shamers needed was something more complicated, something with a lot of math involved, something only an astronomer could dream up. They found it in the work of Adolphe Quetelet. In the 1930s, the Belgian scientist set out to show how the rules of statistics and probability could also be adapted to measure -- even predict! -- human behavior. He collected mounds of height and weight data from a large group of military recruits and plotted the calculated results into, as expected, a bell-shaped curve. Eureka! Quetelet somehow noticed that -- significant or not -- the average weight (in kilograms) of the most "average" soldiers was proportional to their height, (in meters) *squared*. From there, the astronomer went on to argue that an average weight should also be considered the "ideal" weight. This might not seem so sinister if Quetelet was more detached from his work and didn't already believe that criminals and other social deviants could be distinguished by their physical characteristics.[27]

25: Gaesser.
26: Campos, Paul. *The Obesity Myth.* New York: Gotham Books. 2004.
27: Oliver, J. Eric. *Fat Politics: The Real Story Behind America's Obesity Epidemic.* New York: Oxford University Press, 2006

Looking to improve on the simple height-weight charts popularized by MetLife, fat-fighters in the 1950s returned to the Belgian's formula and gave it added traction, describing it as a measure of "Body Mass Index," or BMI. To make the original metric system formula work with the Americans' messy measures of pounds and inches, mathletes came up with the mystical multiplier of 703. And it looked like this:

BMI = Weight (in pounds) divided by height (in inches, squared), multiplied by 703.

To find your BMI using your pocket Candy Crush device, find the calculator app and, when no one is looking, enter: (your weight in pounds) ÷ (your height in inches) ÷ (height in inches, again) ✕ 703. If you did it right, you'll have a two-digit number left of the decimal point.

For perspective, you may prefer an antique BMI chart. It's interesting to see where your height and weight stats align on the grid, especially if you're little square abuts the dividing line between those seemingly arbitrary classifications. If only you could drop six or seven pounds (or grow an inch), you think, then you'd be in that nice category with those nice people weighing 25 or 30 pounds less than you do. Despite being a poor measure of obesity and a worse measure of health, BMI measurements have become pervasive, not only in popular culture but as a cornerstone of public health policy. History now recognizes 1988 as the year of the BMI Apocalypse. In a single day, 37 million Americans of average weight awoke to being classified as overweight for the first time.

This was not the day after Thanksgiving. It was the day the U.S. National Institutes of Health, in order to fall in line with the stricter standards of the World Health Organization, abandoned its overweight threshold of BMI 27.8 for men and 27.3 for women. Since that time, both men and women in the U.S. have been considered overweight at BMI 25 and up, or obese at BMI 30.[28] Additionally, BMIs of 35, 40 and 50 are customarily said to delineate the gateway to being labeled "severely," "morbidly" and "super" obese.

Imagine how the whole debate would flip if the descriptors were changed to "successfully obese," "boldly obese" and "courageously obese."

28: Oliver.

But it still wouldn't matter. Regardless of where the artificial boundaries are drawn, *the relationship between individual weight and specific health concerns remains largely one of association, not causation.*

Men with typical male pattern baldness are 36 percent more likely to have heart disease. That's a true fact.[29] But no one is suggesting baldness *causes* heart disease. Calculations of Body Mass Index can be equally misleading, especially for athletes, women, and children. For one thing, that factor of 703 in the BMI formula has the effect of smoothing out pesky variables like age, gender and height. And BMI is clearly clumsy when attempting to distinguish fat from lean muscle tissue. Individual variances in water weight, bone and cartilage are bulldozed under by the averaging process.

APPLES AND PEARS

BMI calculations imply that all fat is bad. We know better.

Fat cushions and protects our bones and organs. It insulates the body and protects it from cold. And it stores energy better than any battery contemplated for the next generation of electric vehicles. Recognize also that fat itself is one of the body's most complex organs, receiving and transmitting life-sustaining information and producing regulatory hormones such as leptin and resistin.

But there is one type of adipose tissue that will continue to give fat a bad name. It's the deep visceral fat including the glop that globs around internal organs. Too much of it reveals itself as the characteristic apple shape, most commonly in men. And even though "excess weight" alone has been unfairly blamed for all manner of health problems, there is -- I flatly concede -- compelling evidence that visceral fat is associated with a higher risk of conditions leading to diabetes and heart disease.

It's the type of tissue that releases fats into the bloodstream, lards ups your liver, and mucks up your metabolism. It has been linked to raising levels of bad cholesterol, lowering good cholesterol, and promoting insulin resistance. Visceral fat feeds on bad habits, including stress and smoking and, of course, fatty foods, sweets and alcohol. Some men and women with potbellies are familiar with such indulgences.

29: Sigh. I miss the pre-"fake news" era when all facts were true.

Good news! Visceral fat is the first to respond to regular exercise. This doesn't mean "spot" exercise. Sit-ups, for example, will strengthen stomach muscles, but they do not target stomach fat. To burn fat, especially visceral fat, the best torch is regular aerobic exercise, e.g. walking, golfing, swimming, jogging, chasing rabbits.

If you're known for your thunder thighs or for packing a lot of junk in the trunk, cut yourself some slack. Not only will you be more comfortable sitting on a hard bench at your kid's softball game or oboe recital, you're probably going to outlive all your skinny friends.

Although apple and pear shapes are easily generalized as beer bellies and bubble butts, there is an easy, inexpensive way to objectively measure fat distribution. Simply use a tape measure to circumnavigate the waist and hips at their fullest positions. Divide the belly number by the butt number and hope for a number less than one.

The World Health Organization and most public health organizations believe a "healthy ratio" is important to protect against heart disease and Type 2 diabetes. For women, the high risk category begins at .86, according to the WHO. Moderate risk falls within .81 to .85; low risk is .80 or less.

So, the classic "hourglass" figure of a woman with a 24-inch waist and 36-inch hips would have a ratio of .66. Take a picture. It'll last longer. In the real world, a woman with 36-inch hips needs a waist no larger than 30.6 inches just to stay in the moderate risk category with a ratio of .85. Other examples of the .85 ratio include waist and hip measurements of 34 and 40, 36 and 42, 40 and 47, 44 and 51.7.

The risk factor for men is more forgiving. High risk ratios begin at 1.0. At least the math is easy: any measurement where the waist circumference is bigger than the hips is labeled high risk. For adult men, a ratio of .95 or less is considered low risk.

Most of us, including a growing percentage of women, will be bigger around the waist. Any ratio above 1 is considered an apple shape and therefore at higher risk than pear people. One study found that abdominal obesity is associated with higher risk for cancer and cardiovascular disease. Waist-to-hip ratios predict cardiovascular problems more reliably than BMI or waist circumference alone, according to another study. Thicker waist measurements also were linked to Type 2 diabetes in another study.[30]

Fertility issues have been examined in the same light. One batch of research concluded that regardless of BMI women topping the .80 threshold have lower pregnancy rates than women with lower ratios. On the plus side, mothers with wide hips (but a low WTH ratio) may give birth to smarter kids because of their higher levels of certain fatty acids which nourish fetal brain development.[31]

Despite arguments that waist-to-hip ratios are more accurate than BMI or waist measurements alone in predicting diseases associated with obesity, the tale of the tape measure has its problems, too.

Men and women of very different heights can have the same waist-to-hip ratio, thereby proving . . . umm, not much? For certain, the ratio test is not meaningful for children, adults shorter than 5 feet tall, or those with a BMI of 35 or higher. The elasticity and exact placement of the tape can skew results. Laymen tend to measure waists at navel height. You know where your belly button is. Experts prefer taking the circumference at the top of the iliac crest. Do you know where that is?

Evidently, it was important enough to be among the issues carefully considered at a four-day World Health Organization conference devoted exclusively to waist circumference and waist-hip ratios. The WHO released a 47-page report for those of us unable to attend the gut / butt summit in Geneva, Switzerland.

Will public health policymakers continue to seek a simplified measurement of human fat as an inexpensive shortcut to personalized, unbiased health diagnosis and treatment? Probably, just as there will continue to be enough exceptions to the rules equating weight with health to keep the concept of an "obesity paradox" alive and well.

For most of us, any struggle to fit into some old jeans is reliable evidence that important bodily changes are taking place. So pay attention.

30: "Waist-to-hip Ratio: How Does It Affect Your Health?" Medicalnewstoday.com. Undated.

31: W. Lassek and S. Gaulin S. "Waist-hip Ratio and Cognitive Ability: Is Gluteofemoral Fat A Privileged Store of Neurodevelopmental Resources?" *Evolution and Human Behavior*. January 2008)

But regardless of whether your belt is inexplicably tight, or where your data dot falls on the BMI scale or waist-to-hip ratio, the health advice is the same: Eat like a bunny and chase more rabbits.

03

PUSHERS

No one *told* you to get fat.

N o one, including me, is suggesting you get fatter.

But dozens of times each day -- sometime hundreds -- you are casually reminded or blatantly encouraged to enjoy all the seemingly addictive things that can make you fat. Billions of dollars in advertising are carefully aimed at children and adults to reinforce a lifelong appetite for highly processed and tempting foods, snacks and drinks. Whether by trust, naivete or subconscious conditioning, we submit to the good-humored recommendations for daylong snacking. And when the time for foods with genuine nutrition arrives? Meh. We're just not that hungry.

Meanwhile, news reports are filled with study after study building the case linking fast food and soft drinks with rising rates of obesity. The calorie industry is not deaf to these warning bells. Thus far, it has mounted a successful defense by offering token compromises, promoting personal freedom and choice, building or buying coalitions with opponents, and making puppy-eyed promises of self-regulation. While the calorie industry succeeds just by leaving the public at large feeling guilty or confused, its lobbyists have turned back all but a few isolated efforts to increase government intervention via sugar taxes or tougher constraints on ads which put children squarely in their line of fire.

From the industry perspective, this whole little misunderstanding about cheap calories, obesity, diabetes, and soaring health care costs is just a matter of lax personal and parental responsibility and, by implication, our puny efforts to resist their well-researched and perniciously packaged marketing.

Without embarrassment, and without accepting any blame, the food giants even fund special sponsorships and promotions to suggest that even though they are not part of the problem, they want to be part of the solution.

One such event took place on a steamy August afternoon on a sun-drenched Florida campus.

The media having dutifully assembled, representatives of a well-known soft drink giant proudly announced a refreshing gift of $1.1 million to assist the University of Gainesville with a pilot program called the Family Health Self-Empowerment Project. In a state where six out of 10 adults are overweight or obese, the university hoped to show it could make a difference, starting with 600 low-income households selected within the local community. Participants in the program would attend five bi-weekly workshops where they would learn about making better food choices and preparing healthier ethnic meals while keeping a journal to document their daily eating, exercise, and television-watching routines.[32]

It takes big money to make a difference in the firmly entrenched habits of the public, as when the National Cancer Institute budgeted $1 million for a "5 A Day" fruits and vegetable serving campaign, or when the National Health, Lung and Blood Institute budgeted $1.5 million for a national cholesterol education campaign.

But in a nation of 300-plus million souls, of which 200 million occupy overweight or obese bodies, Big Soda's gift of a million dollars was little more than a publicity stunt hosted by a major university. The soft drink giant's gift was equal to what it would spend on average every seven hours and five minutes for national advertising during the following year.

Around the time of the Gainesville promotion, the bubble bottler's budget for all forms of advertising was nearly $1.3 billion. That's about $4.39 per American.

32: Diane Chun. "Pepsi Gives $1.1 Million Grant to UF Anti-Obesity Project." August 29, 2006. *www. gainesville.com.*

Major soft drink producers are solid companies with thousands of employees and millions of satisfied investors and customers. But with few exceptions, their product lines are primarily built on what nutritionists politely call empty calories. While paid advertising links their products with youth, fun, friends, health and sex, company executives will tell critics their products are not intended to replace healthier foods. They will say that their perfectly safe snack foods and soft drinks should be enjoyed occasionally, or in moderation and as part of a routine that includes fresh vegetables and exercise. And all that advertising? It's necessary to protect and maybe expand their share of a legal, lucrative and open market.

There are at least 20 corporations in the U.S. that spend more each year on advertising than Coca-Cola and PepsiCo. They are the biggies of consumer products and entertainment, such as Procter & Gamble, Verizon, General Motors, Time-Warner, GlaxoSmithKline, Bank of America, Sears and Sony.

Countless studies have linked the supersizing of Americans to easy access to empty calories. And even if most corporations have their frequent critics and occasional P.R. meltdowns, the Teflon resilience of today's obesity profiteers is second only to the persistence of the tobacco industry.

IN THE CROSSHAIRS

Advertisements for food permeate television, radio, magazines, the internet and mobile media. Scattershot marketing is limited to the Super Bowl and a few billboards. The greatest bulk of spending goes to carefully identified subgroups such as care-free singles, work-weary adults, picky children, nagged parents, and massive ethnic "minority" groups.

Does it work? The same media executives who say prime time television's lust for sex and violence has no adverse influence on audience behavior will sing a completely different tune when it's time to sign up advertisers for a pricey 30 seconds of air time. Advertisers sift through audience and reader demographics like miners panning for gold nuggets, then spend millions more testing their messages on focus groups. Then comes the real money -- billions for ads to put the research into motion, each dollar of it finely chiseled to pierce its target segment, be it families, men, women, seniors, adults, whites, blacks, Hispanics, teens, tweens, children or preschoolers.

Consumers riddled by guilt over their food and beverage choices may as well accept blame for being human, being hungry and having eyes and ears to absorb the bombardment of messages urging consumption of the sweetest, saltiest and fattest foods, all of them affordable and within easy reach.

One market research group estimates that a person living in a city will see as many as 5,000 advertising messages a day, up from a measly 2,000 a day 30 years ago. No, they're not all for fast food and soft drinks, but there are enough of them to push apples and bananas far off the consciousness radar.

Add to that the most persuasive marketing of all -- the ubiquitous availability of snack foods and soft drinks placed at eye level and within arm's reach. You know from experience that 95 percent of drug stores and gas stations devote generous shelf space to snack foods. It's no longer unusual for general merchandise stores and even those specializing in clothing, hardware, books, garden supplies or auto parts to make it ultra-convenient to pick up extra calories during the day. And these are calories we will not remember to compensate for when an actual meal time rolls around.[33]

Strip away the detail and brand names, and all advertising is designed to sell envy -- not so much of the neighbors or the Joneses, but of a future self that is just one more purchase away from satisfaction and happiness, whether it's a purse and matching shoes, the next-generation game console or an easily affordable stack of hamburger, bacon and cheese.

Most of us grip our wallets tightly when faced with a sales pitch for a life insurance or a new roof and gutters. But the marketers of fast food and sugary drinks have it easy. Their products are inexpensive and still have high profit margins. Their goodies are intended for consumption the moment the cash register rings, and can be quickly replaced when hunger returns. One more big advantage: these delicious products can affect brain chemistry in the same ways drugs and alcohol create dependence.

ADDICTED TO FOOD

It doesn't take a rocket scientist to boost flavors with sugars, salt and fat. That secret has been around as long as honey and butter. Nevertheless, modern

33: "Does Junk Food at Non-Food Stores Add Pounds?" Reuters Health. January 11, 2010.

food processors and marketers maintain a standing army of food scientists to tweak the taste balance of their products as they move from test kitchens to focus groups and on to 24/7 sales. Whether it's intentional or not, those added flavors and textures may create addiction-like responses.

In a study of 350 Yale undergraduates -- a group we'd all like to think is reasonably intelligent and self-aware -- 11 percent of respondents met the standard mental disorder definition of substance dependence, based solely on their relationship with foods. In particular, many reported a loss of control when eating, a persistent desire or effort to cut back, and repeated use despite negative consequences.[34]

Researchers were surprised when they found very obese people had lower levels of dopamine in the reward areas of their brains than did people of normal weight. Previously, the Conventional Wisdom was that people who become addicted to drugs (or food) were releasing more pleasure-inducing dopamine. Now we know the opposite effect is more likely. People who don't get a normal dopamine response from food or drugs want more, more, more because they're less easily satisfied.

Are some people destined to overeat because they were born with sluggish dopamine response? Or does overeating over-stimulate and eventually dampen the reward mechanism? Yes and yes, ongoing research suggests. In one experiment, a group of young overweight and obese women began and ended a six-month evaluation by having their dopamine response measured while enjoying a chocolate milkshake. The ones who had gained weight during the six months had a lower dopamine response than those who gained no weight.

"Just as drug addicts use more to chase their original high, obese individuals may need to eat more food to compensate for these changes," said Cara Bohon, a researcher at the University of California, Los Angeles.[35]

In another study, researchers found that blah, blah, blah . . .

Hey! Eyes on the page! You're still thinking about that sweet, creamy milkshake, aren't you? The best way to lose interest in that shake is to have one,

---

34: Bonnie Liebman. "Food and Addiction: Can Some Foods Hijack the Brain?" Nutrition Action Newsletter. May 1, 2012.
35: Devin Powell, Inside News Service. "Milkshake Like Cocaine for Overeaters." *livescience.com.* September 29, 2010.

and then you'll lose interest well before your satiety hormones kick in. The study I was trying to tell you about showed greater activity in the brain while subjects merely *looked at a picture of a milkshake* than when they were actually drinking one.

Food porn! It's hot! It's real. Kids like it, too! And your brain loves the extended foreplay so much that temptation is hard to resist.

THE INCREDIBLE CRAVEABLE OREO

Addiction is not a word casually bandied in the boardrooms or public pronouncements of America's major snack food producers. They still haven't forgotten how tobacco executives testified in 1994 before Congress and God (representing, I think, two extremes on the integrity continuum) that nicotine was *not* addictive. When several of the millions of internal documents later surrendered to the courts proved otherwise, the unartful dodge cost the tobacco industry hundreds of billions of dollars in liability claims.

In 2005, the *Chicago Tribune* published a sprawling, immaculately documented series called "The Oreo, Obesity and Us." In it, the links between foods, marketing, addiction and obesity were carefully detailed.

It was a gutsy display of independent journalism, considering the hometown connection. You see, Nabisco's bakery in Chicago (where 600 jobs were recently exported to Mexico) was then the largest in the world, with 1,500 employees churning out 320 million pounds of snack foods a year. Nabisco's corporate history is equally intriguing, given its association with the tobacco industry. Nabisco merged with R.J. Reynolds in 1985 and was acquired in 2000 by Philip Morris Companies, Inc., which then merged Nabisco with Kraft Foods. Fortunately, this did not lead to the marketing of Cheesy Marlboros or Menthol Oreos. Nevertheless, as documents later revealed, the mergers did encourage cooperation between staff scientists from the tobacco and snack food companies. In one such example, a Kraft researcher (whose doctorate in neuroscience included studies on obesity, rats and hunger-blocking opiate drugs) organized meetings between Kraft's own brain scientists and their peers at Philip Morris who were studying the effects of nicotine.[36]

36: Jeremy Manier, Patricia Callahan and Delroy Alexander. "The Oreo, Obesity and Us: Craving the Cookie." *Chicago Tribune*. August 21, 2005.

Other documents sifted out by the *Chicago Tribune* show a reciprocal interest from a nicotine researcher at Philip Morris who discussed the possibility of collaborative studies that would be of "mutual interest" to Kraft and the tobacco group.

For the record, a Kraft spokeswoman said the company had studied thousands of aspects of food science, especially regarding which flavors and smells appeal to consumers, but denied the company sponsored any research "aimed at creating consumer dependency upon any of our products." [37]

And yet creating a "betcha-can't-eat-just-one" formula is exactly what drives food processing research, according to some former insiders.

Bill Bradley spent 15 years overseeing some best-known brands of Nabisco, Pillsbury and General Mills, but became increasingly uncomfortable with his role in the industry before leaving. Now he writes a blog that is often critical of trends in the food industry.

"I decided to step out and ultimately speak out in hopes of bringing more awareness to the issue," he told Canadian journalist Kelly Crowe. "What we eat and drink from a lot of these big food and beverages companies isn't that good for us. These products are designed to keep you coming back to eat more and more and more." [38]

When Bradley says "product," he really means product. "We're not talking about food actually being real anymore. It's synthetic, completely contrived and created, and there's so many problems about that because our bodies are tricked. And when our bodies are tricked repeatedly, dramatic things can happen -- like weight gain."

Behind the commercial images of carefree kids and sugar-fueled teens enjoying fresh air, exercise, sunshine and colorfully-packaged snack foods and sweet drinks, food scientists are working hard in well-equipped laboratories to find the best ratio of chewiness, crunch, sweetness, saltiness, fat balance and overall "mouth feel." They search for the exact "bliss point" by adding just enough sweetener, but no more. Technicians and trained tasters will be on guard for "sensory specific satiety" -- a flavor, or even a texture that is *too* satisfying for

---

37: Manier and others. *Chicago Tribune.*
38: Kelly Crowe. "Food Cravings Engineered By Industry." March 6, 2013. cbc.ca.

extended snacking. Instead, they make tiny adjustments to achieve "vanishing caloric density," with flavors and textures that disappear in the mouth faster than the brain registers the intake of calories. They measure the intensity of a crunch and how well it travels through the jaw bones, knowing each sound helps to keep customer engaged and eating.[39]

The jargon of engineered craving and much more are revealed in Michael Moss's stomach-churning expose, *Salt Sugar Fat: How the Food Giants Hooked Us*. The Pulitzer winner writer had been investigating a surge in deadly outbreaks of E. coli in meat when an industry source suggested that he explore an even bigger public health hazard. Find out, the microbiologist urged, what food companies were *intentionally* adding to their products.[40]

"It's not just a matter of poor willpower on the part of the consumer and a give-the-people-what-they-want attitude on the part of the food manufacturers," Moss says. "What I found, over four years of research and reporting, was a conscious effort. . . to get people hooked on foods that are convenient and inexpensive." [41]

Food processors also devote a lot of research and energy to lowering the cost of production and extending shelf life. Those same modifications can replace pleasant tastes with bad flavors or a bland overlap of competing tones. The solution? Add more salt, sugar or fats along with other chemical enhancers to make the products not just palatable, but irresistible. Several independent studies have shown how sweet, rich foods cause the brain to release pleasure-inducing opiates similar to those created in a drug-related high. Or, as yet another study found, the same drugs used in blocking the appeal of opiates can also make sweets less appealing.

"Salt, sugar and fat are the pillars of the processed food industry," Moss says. "And while the industry hates the word 'addiction' more than any other word, the fact of the matter is their research has shown them that when they hit the perfect amounts of each of those ingredients. . . they will have us buy more, eat more."[42]

39: Crowe.
40: Michael Moss. *Salt Sugar Fat: How the Food Giants Hooked Us*. Random House. 2013.
41: Kelly Crowe. Michael Moss quoted in "Food Cravings Engineered by Industry: How Big Food Keeps Us Eating Through a Combination of Science and Marketing." March 23, 2013. *CBC News*.
42: Crowe.

The psychology and physiology of food addiction may be a dark science to researchers, but millions of self-described food junkies have found solace in being open about their battle with habituation. Since 1960, the 12-step program used by Overeaters Anonymous has been effective using the same blunt honesty and group support techniques embraced by recovering alcoholics, drug abusers, and gamblers.

CHILDREN KNOW WHAT $4.6 BILLION LOOKS LIKE

Given the addictively flavored ingredients, low cost, ready availability and unavoidable advertising for fast food and soft drinks, it's not surprising how many adults are wearing the new calorie culture around their waists.

Now, try rearing hungry, growing, picky, mobile and easily persuaded children in this same environment. The closest thing to a surprise is that *only* one in three children in America is overweight or obese. We are left to assume the millions of kids are sneaking in vigorous exercise each day just by texting, fidgeting on the couch, swinging a Wii remote, skateboarding or walking two miles to Bojangles.

And that's a good thing, because the reach and impact of calories marketed to children begins at age two and never lets up.

In 2012 the fast food industry spent $4.6 billion to advertise mostly unhealthy products. Children and teens were the key audiences for that advertising, according to an exhaustive report by the Yale Rudd Center for Food Policy & Obesity. Compared to a baseline study conducted two years prior, the report was able to find only a few positive developments, such as healthier sides and beverages in most restaurants' kids' meals.[43]

"There were some improvements, but they have been small, and the pace too slow," said Marlene Schwartz, Rudd Center director. "Without more significant changes, we are unlikely to see meaningful reductions in unhealthy fast food consumption by young people."

The most recent report, "Fast Food FACTS 2013," was presented at an annual meeting of the American Public Health Association. It examined 18

43: "Fast Food FACTS 2013." Rudd Center for Food Policy & Obesity.

of the top fast-food restaurants in the United States and documented changes in the nutritional quality of menu items along with changes in marketing to children and teens on TV, the Internet, social media, and mobile devices. The report was supported by a grant from the Robert Wood Johnson Foundation. I mention that to help assure you these are actual fact-based facts, not alternative facts or a baseless rant.

Among the important findings:

Children ages 6 to 11 saw 10 percent fewer TV ads for fast food, but children and teens continued to see three to five fast food ads on TV every day.

Healthier kids' meals were advertised by a few restaurants, but they represented only one-quarter of fast-food ads viewed by children.

Less than 1 percent of kids' meals combinations at restaurants met nutrition standards recommended by experts, and just 3 percent met the industry's own back-patting standards touted as the Children's Food and Beverage Advertising Initiative and Kids LiveWell nutrition standards.

Spanish-language advertising to Hispanic preschoolers, a population at high risk for obesity, increased by 16%.

Fast food marketing via social media and mobile devices — media that are popular with teens — grew exponentially.

McDonald's led the way with $971.8 million in total advertising in 2012, according to the Rudd Center's analysis of Nielsen data. TV spending consumed nearly 80 percent of that, but still left more than $86 million *each* for radio and outdoor advertising and $6.6 million for internet promotions.[44]

Subway was the second biggest spender in 2012 with $595.3 in total -- a 39 percent jump from 2009. Taco Bell and Wendy's each contributed about $275 million to our nutrition education, followed by KFC, Pizza Hut, Burger King, Domino's, Sonic and Papa John's, where $153.3 million was only good enough for 10th place.[45]

44: "Fast Food FACTS 2013." Rudd Center for Food Policy & Obesity.
45: "Fast Food FACTS 2013." Rudd Center for Food Policy & Obesity.

What does all that buy? A lot of little eyeballs. Preschoolers, age 2-5 years, saw an average of 1,024 fast food ads on national, cable, and local TV during 2012 -- just a little shy of the 1,175 ads reaching children age 6-11. McDonald's -- no surprise -- had the most impressions, reaching preschoolers 265 times in a one year, plus 316 times for older kids.

Mothers need not wonder why so many of their children's whines begin with "Mommmm, take us to...."

"Most fast food restaurants stepped up advertising to children and teens," said Jennifer Harris, the Rudd Center's director of marketing initiatives and lead author of the report. "Most advertising promotes unhealthy regular menu items and often takes unfair advantage of young people's vulnerability to marketing, making it even tougher for parents to raise healthy children."[46]

The authors recommended that restaurants apply nutrition standards to all kids' meals and automatically provide healthy sides and beverages, rather than defaulting to fries and soft drinks. They also should stop marketing their least healthy items to children and teens in ways that take advantage of their vulnerabilities, the researchers said.

Recommendations aren't law. And there is not a snow cone's chance in a pizza oven of new advertising restraints with business-friendly lawmakers dominating Washington and most statehouses.

Parents who aren't able to limit their children's exposure to inappropriate advertising will have to make their stand in their kitchens. Preparing healthy meals and snacks doesn't take any more effort than following a trail of tail lights inching toward a carryout window.

46: "Fast Food FACTS 2013." Rudd Center for Food Policy & Obesity.

04

DO JEAN'S GENES MAKE HER LOOK FAT?

Your tight jeans are talking about you behind your back. They tell us there is an ample supply of fat stored in your body tissue. They reflect that there are generous and readily available reserves of calories awaiting your selection in the refrigerator, in the pantry, and at restaurants and food markets just short drives away.

Your metabolic genes hold the keys to storing fat or converting it to energy. But they don't know when you're likely to eat again. Will it be five minutes? Or five days? Even longer? Funny how they are smart enough to remember back hundreds, even millions, of years, but can't see five seconds into the future.

If only Jean could get through to Gene. "Can't you see we have plenty to eat," Jean would scream, bursting a double-stitched seam. "We could be burning more carbs to make some extra energy around here -- *now*. Enough with stockpiling fat. There's not going to be a famine! Okay?"

Still, Jean should give Gene more credit. What if Jean is injured, in a coma, and unable to eat for weeks? Or she gets lost in the woods and can't stomach a *Fear Factor* diet of twigs and squishy things until the search team arrives? Even in a land of plenty, a personal famine could be just around the corner for any of us. Such emergencies are rare, admittedly, but heft, as much as attitude, is often what determines whether your life story is headlined "Survivor" or "Obituary."

Whatever. For most of us, how we *look* in a pair of jeans is what's important today and a hundred tomorrows. Pity the pants. They have to stretch enough to contain rumps with more rolls than a French bakery, along with all the emotional baggage of weight-related guilt, insecurity, stigma, blame, and self-loathing. Genetics and the obesogenic environment be damned, the individual's duty to muster more restraint has always dominated the obesity discussion. It was even institutionalized in 2004 when the U.S. House of Representatives passed legislation hailed as the Personal Responsibility in Food Consumption Act. Similar to laws already considered in several states, the so-called Cheeseburger Bill was drafted in response to a flurry of lawsuits against McDonald's and other fast-food restaurants by plump patrons who blamed the chains for serving up all that addictively fat and delicious food.

I would say the litigation and legislation were both overkill. I want to believe hunches and hysteria about obesity will eventually give way to hard science, including the dozens of studies referenced in this book.

METABOLISM

We all have family members and co-workers with the annoying ability to seemingly eat whatever they want, whenever they want, without gaining weight and without spending evenings at the gym. Gee-darn their washboard stomachs! And many of us have known of a young athlete or long-time jogger whose life was abruptly ended by heart attack or disease. Surely, inherited or congenital traits must be a contributing factor.

Still, many health experts cling to the faux maxim that being overweight can only come from consuming more food energy than is expended in activity. Purely as physics, the equation makes perfect sense. Individually, however, our complicated bodies are making their own rules about how much energy is spent, and how much is deposited in the fat bank.

"Scientists have found that our genes not only determine our natural weight range, but they also determine our energy levels, feelings of hunger and satiation, and the ways our bodies absorb sugar and fat."[47] The words are those of J. Eric Oliver. He made a deep dive into the obesity blame game in his 2006 book, *Fat Politics.*

And this, from a study by Jeffrey M. Friedman and Jeffrey L. Halaas into

---

47: Oliver, J. Eric, *Fat Politics*, Oxford University Press, 2006.

the impact of the hormone *leptin* on body weight in mammals: "The belief that obesity is largely the result of a lack of willpower, though widely held, is unsatisfactory." Studies of twins adopted and raised separately and animal models of obesity "all indicate that obesity is the result of both genetic and environmental factors."[48]

Read that again, and instantly shed a few more pounds of guilt. It means that try as we might to make adjustments in our eating and exercise habits, the body's internal blueprint will pull us back toward the house that Gene built.

Those who study biology and metabolism in the context of evolution have found a strong scientific basis for what is called the *thrifty gene hypothesis*. Food scarcity being the norm throughout most of history, the ability to store energy reserves during times of abundance was an undeniable advantage. Those who were able to store fat survived and reproduced; those who looked svelte in a loincloth were less likely to thrive and pass on their genetic traits.

That ability to invest fat for the future correlates with genetic influence on individual metabolic rates. Any prolonged effort to alter these innate body rhythms will be met with resistance, as 41 human lab rats experienced during a carefully monitored 1995 study at Rockefeller University's Laboratory of Human Behavior and Metabolism.[49]

Starting with a test group of 18 obese patients and 23 others who had never been obese, the scientists carefully monitored every calorie consumed and measured their energy expended around the clock whether resting or active. A little refresher class for those of you who were nodding off in Biology 102: Physical activity for humans accounts for only about 30 percent of total energy expenditures. Another 10 percent is the thermic, or warming effect, of digestion and transporting nutrients. The remaining 60 percent of our energy is spent even while resting. And no, we can't double our couch time to burn twice the calories.

After ascertaining each test subject's baseline values, the investigators dramatically increased or reduced individual caloric intake for several months,

---

48: Friedman, Jeffrey M., and Jeffrey L. Halaas, *"Leptin And The Regulation of Body Weight in Mammals,"* Nature 395, 763-770, October 22, 1998.
49: Leibel, Rudolph L., M.D.,and otheretpoint. *"Changes in Energy Expenditure Resulting from Altered Body Weight,"* The New England Journal of Medicine. March 9, 2005.

until everyone either gained or lost 10 percent of their original weight. Because the test volunteers all lived at the laboratory and were subject to continuous observation (again, like rats), scientists were able to observe and record all activities. And here's what they found:

- Those who were given more calories and gained 10 percent of their weight became more fidgety, burning more calories even during rest periods. Careful measurements showed that, on average, they were expending 16 percent more total energy in a 24-hour period.

- Those on restricted-calorie diets appeared more tranquil as their bodies adjusted to the forced starvation. Measurements confirmed the observations. A 10 percent weight loss resulted in a 15 percent reduction in energy expenditures.

The conclusion of the study, as reported in the New England Journal of Medicine: "Maintenance of a reduced or elevated body weight is associated with compensatory changes in energy expenditure, which oppose the maintenance of a body weight that is different from the usual body weight."[50]

Researchers even said these unconscious adjustments in energy management may explain the long-term failure of so-called treatments for obesity. Unfortunately, it seems personal metabolism is a fit opponent for any amount of willpower and will outsmart the most ingenious weight-loss scheme. One unsurprising footnote: This study has since been cited by literally a hundred other scientific studies but is consistently ignored in the sales pitches delivered by the best-known diet or fitness programs. Other studies, including several involving family members or pairs of twins have also supported the theory of *homeostasis* — the body's natural tendency to maintain and defend its natural weight. Whether that *set point* for an individual's weight is high or low or varies over a wide range seems to be largely an inherited trait.[51]

A 2005 study published by researchers at the nutrition and genomics laboratory at Tufts University also identified a genetic variant in the *perilipin* proteins which play a role in the conversion of body fat to energy. The genetic deviation appears to strengthen the body's normal efforts to maintain

---

50: Leibel and others.
51: Oliver.

homeostasis. Although an earlier study had linked the gene with a lower rate of obesity, the follow-up also revealed it can make some people more resistant to losing weight by cutting calories.

"It may make sense," said Andrew Greenberg, M.D., director of the Tufts research center, "if we consider that this perilipin gene variant induces a sort of *buffer* against changes in how the body burns and stores food energy. It appears to protect against weight gain in lean women, while preventing weight loss in men and women who have become obese," Greenberg said when the findings were announced.[52]

And here's another fetching finding from researchers at the University of California, San Francisco, who managed to locate and study 28 pairs of identical, male twins where one brother was a regular runner and the other more sedentary. Without altering their exercise habits, the pairs were put on either a high-fat or low-fat diet. After six weeks, all participants switched to the other diet. By flip-flopping the lifestyle variables, the study appeared to show that genetics — not diet or exercise — had the strongest effect on blood cholesterol.[53]

HORMONE HIJINKS

Other areas of study have identified specific hormones, acids and proteins -- all with genetic influence -- which challenge even the strongest willpower for control of our appetites. You are doubtless familiar with the guttural impact of *ghrelin*, a hormone produced in the stomach. Levels vary throughout the day, and are highest as meal times approach. Hungry? Then you're gellin' with ghrelin. A genetically transmitted surplus of ghrelin also may explain why some people are challenged by hunger that is virtually uncontrollable.

In 1994, researchers discovered a critical component among the body's weight-management tools. The leptin hormone is produced within fat tissues and notifies the brain when fat reserves are sufficient to reduce appetite. That's good. The bad news: Over time, our bodies become less receptive to leptin's

---

52: "Nutritional Genomics Identifies a Potential Weight-loss Resistance Gene." News release, Friedman School of Nutrition Science and Policy at Tufts University. December 7, 2005.
53: Woznicki, Katrina, "Twin Study Shows Genes Have Major Clout Over Cholesterol Levels," MedPage Today, July 8, 2005, a teaching brief, peer-reviewed by University of Pennsylvania School of Medicine.

message. Normally, a rapid gain in weight is rapidly lost. But in some cases, Friedman reported, the increase of leptin levels during weight gain leads to a reduction in body's response to leptin and "a failure to return to the starting weight."[54] This cycle of increased leptin production and neural resistance also explains why efforts to treat obesity with leptin injections have been ineffective in most test subjects.

So feel free to tell anyone insensitive to your weight battles that you, too, are being insensitive — to leptin.

Conventional wisdom also has long held that obesity contributes to *insulin resistance* and Type 2 diabetes. But here, too, new findings about the role of genetics require an open mind.

Back to basics first. The carbohydrates we eat are either converted in our bodies to sugars for energy or stored as fat. Certain foods, such as pure sugars and refined carbohydrates, are said to have a high *glycemic load* because they are easily converted to glucose, resulting in a spike in blood sugar levels. As blood sugar rises, the pancreas produces more insulin to round up the glucose and escort it to the waiting cells. The energy that comes with a "sugar high" doesn't last long. Feeling pooped and hungry, the body craves another glycemic fix, and too often we oblige it with more junk calories.

Over time, the body becomes annoyed by the sugar peaks and valleys and its sugar-rich cells become less responsive to absorbing glucose. The pancreas, however, doesn't get the memo about the work stoppage at the loading dock, and produces more insulin to deal with the backup in glucose delivery. Finally, the pancreas is exhausted and refuses to produce enough insulin to handle even the small deliveries of glucose. In medical circles, this cluster-fudge is called Type 2 diabetes. Left untreated, the disease can cause blindness and the kind of circulatory problems that literally cost an arm or a leg, or an early death.

These are all good reasons to give yourself half a chance to avoid insulin resistance by exercising and eating right. I say "half" because researchers now believe that genetics determines almost half of an individual's variability in insulin action, the rest being determined by diet, fitness and other lifestyle factors.

54: Friedman.

Evidence of the genetic contribution to insulin resistance came from studying different groups chosen for their lack of diversity such as families or close-knit tribes of Native Americans. The mounting evidence shows that insulin resistance is greater among American Indians, African-Americans and Mexican-Americans, as well as Australian Aboriginals, South Asian Indians and certain Pacific Island groups.

"The results of these studies of individuals, families and large population groups all suggested that genes play a major role in the development of insulin resistance, and that people of non-European ancestry are more likely to have the offending genes," Stanford University endocrinologist Gerald Reaven, M.D.,

writes in his book, *Syndrome X: Overcoming the Silent Killer That Can Give You a Heart Attack.*[55] Reaven says the ability of insulin to do its job can vary tenfold in apparently healthy people.

Differences are likely a complex set of genetic factors, he says, and may result from many combinations of genes. The author also believes that as many as 75 million Americans, even though they are not diabetic, are greatly at risk of coronary heart disease because of damage to blood vessels caused by insulin resistance.

Since the time Reaven's work was published, researchers in Iceland have identified a specific gene variant with a clear link to Type 2 diabetes. The link was found by analyzing genetic records of Icelanders, and confirmed with Danish and European-American study groups.

Research continues. For now, fat folks can take comfort in the words of University of Cambridge endocrinologist Dr. Stephen O'Rahilly. "What recent research has done," he says, "is take obesity out of the realm of sociology and put it in the realm of biology."[56]

Right on.

55: Gerald Reaven, M.D., and others, "Syndrome X: Overcoming the Silent Killer That Can Give You a Heart Attack." Simon & Schuster, New York, 2000.

56: Jeffrey Kluger. "Obesity: Healthy Genes Could Mean Smaller Jeans." TIME Magazine, January 15, 2001. Copyright 2006.

RACE, GENDER, AND AGE

Even in an age of heightened political correctness and the success of white hip hop stars such as Eminem and Macklemore, I think we can all agree that race is still a genetically transmitted characteristic. The genetic links between race and obesity are less well known, although there is ample documentation of specific diseases and weight characteristics that are more commonly found in some ethnicities. Even then, gender often trumps race as a predictor.

We know from several studies, for example, that Europeans and their descendant Americans are at higher risk for dementia, skin cancers, multiple sclerosis and coronary artery disease, while African-Americans are a greater risk for hypertension, stroke, kidney failure, and obesity (especially among women).

Will you be as heavy a year from now as you are today? Short of losing a limb or temporarily sweating off a few ounces of dewy freshness, it's a good bet that you will be. Our weight today, even more reliably than genes or gender, is the most reliable of all internal predictors. A flurry of recent studies confirms that prenatal development and every stage of childhood is critical in shaping eating, exercise, and weight patterns as an adult.

A study published in the *British Medical Journal* followed 5,863 kids for five years and found that a lifetime of extra weight was well-established by age 11, especially among black girls.

It's never too early to get it right with child nutrition. There is, however, time to get it wrong -- even in the first week of life, says Dr. Nicolas Stettler, a pediatric nutrition specialist at The Children's Hospital of Philadelphia. His research team found that formula-fed babies who gained weight rapidly during their first week of life were significantly more likely to be overweight decades later. The researcher (who recommends breastfeeding) told Reuters that each additional 3.5 ounces of weight gained during the first eight days of life increased a baby's risk of becoming an overweight adult by about 10 percent.[57]

Even Week One may be considered late intervention for a newborn. A child's weight through at least age 7 may already have been influenced by the mother's weight even before she became pregnant. That's one of the findings in

---

57: Author unknown, "First Week Critical in Childhood Obesity – U.S. Study," April 18, 2005, © Reuters 2005.

a study of more than 3,000 children and their mothers by nursing professors at Ohio State University. A child is also at a greater risk of becoming overweight if he is born to a mother who smoked during her pregnancy, according to the study, which was funded by the National Institutes of Health.

"Weight persists with time, so a child who is overweight by her second birthday is more likely to be overweight at a later age," said Pamela Salsberry, the study's lead author. Rather than blaming genetically transmitted traits, however, Salsberry pointed to evidence linking adult obesity to eating habits formed early in life.[58]

There are still scientists who contend the genetic contribution to obesity is in the range of only 2 to 5 percent. Perhaps they are not factoring in the basic thrifty gene theory that we are all designed to prepare for famine, or the individual genetic contributions to metabolism, appetite, energy conversion and insulin resistance. But the evidence keeps coming. In 2015, the University of Michigan Health System released a new study looking for clues directly related to the BMI of over a half million individuals. They found 97 distinct sites across the human genome -- three times as many as were previously known -- that may influence body weight.[59]

Meanwhile, research into the 20,000-plus genes comprising the human genome continues at a fantastic pace, raising the possibility that we will one day be able to prevent or treat the gamut of our emotional and physical shortcomings -- even gluttony and obesity. But to what extent should we be willing to blame our unhealthy habits on our DNA? Do we put personal responsibility on hold until scientists come up with a "cure" for three trips through a steakhouse buffet? And are we consistent? Do we accept a scientific consensus when it conflicts with personal beliefs about what makes a person smart or stupid, straight or gay, introverted or just pleasantly Fat, Smart and Happy?

I don't have to get famed astrophysicist Neil deGrasse Tyson on the telephone to know what he'd say. "The good thing about science," he reminds children, adults, and childish politicians at every opportunity, "is that it's true

58: "Material Obesity Before Pregnancy Linked to Childhood Weight Problems," Nov. 29, 2005 news release, Ohio State University.
59: "Largest Ever Genome-Wide Study Strengthens Genetic Link to Obesity." uofmhealth.org. (University of Michigan) Feb. 11, 2015. Also, "Genetic Studies of Body Mass Index Yield New Insights for Obesity Biology." Nature. Feb. 11, 2015.

whether or not you believe in it."

Millions of us have studied our own resistance to losing weight. Add that personal experience to the hard science about hormones and metabolism and most adults should find reason enough to forgive their pasts, accept their present and look forward to the future. Obesity trends will not be reversed quickly. Expect the same, slow generational changes that brought us to here and now.

The turning point begins with a mandate for parents and mothers-to-be -- with support from lawmakers, educators, food processors and calorie marketers -- to accept complete responsibility for the emotional and nutritional welfare of children. No matter how it is formulated or measured, a taste of early prevention will go down easier than any remedy available later in life.

05

IT'S A FAT, FAT WORLD

I know how you spent most of your day yesterday. It involved a lot of driving or sitting and reading and screen time and eating and drinking. I'm not being judgy. That's just the world we live in.

Our genetic history continues to respect our long history as hunters and gatherers of the most calorie-rich foods. But the last century of rapid technological advances in growing, processing, and distributing a bounty of delicious foods has obliterated the traditional imbalance of hunger and available calories.

A Conventional Wisdom that might have carried water in simpler times held that animals have an innate sense of nutritional priorities and will select wisely from a wide variety of available foods. A test with lab rats showed that was true when the subjects were provided equally portioned cups of protein, fat, and carbohydrates.

But rats, like humans, can resist everything but temptation. When the researchers gave some of the rats doubled portions of one of the three nutrients, only the subjects offered extra protein continued to thrive. The tests were aborted in just eight days because the rats that switched themselves to a high-fat or high-carb diet had become seriously malnourished from gorging on those energy-dense foods.

A follow-up experiment with liquid calories gave the rodents a choice of plain water or water sweetened with varying amounts of sugar. With a surplus of calories available, and no peer pressure to discourage them, the rats got fat. So much for theories of innate nutritional wisdom.[60]

Now, replace the laboratory in the experiments cited above with the front entrance to a shopping mall. Line it with affordable restaurants serving monstrous portions of pizza, burgers, French fries and soft drinks.

Then substitute you, the motoring public, for the rats in the study, and compare the results. Or look at dozens of similar studies, and you'll reach the same conclusions Yale University nutritionist Dr. Kelly D. Brownell did in researching *Food Fight*, his solution-packed 2004 book about obesity trends: Animals and humans are drawn naturally to an energy-dense diet, he says, and therefore seek out sugar and fat, variety, and flavors associated with fat and carbohydrates.

"Genes cannot adapt quickly enough," Brownell says, "and while we wait for evolution to take its course, humans are locked into a biology that responds poorly to the modern environment."[61]

The insanely rich food environment is now well into its third generation. It began innocently enough. In the mid-1970s, U.S. corn production was soaring and food producers were taking a closer look at the 1971 discovery by Japanese food scientists who devised an economical way to convert truckloads of corn into tanker loads of sweetener. The new high-fructose corn syrup (HFCS) was inexpensive and six times sweeter than cane sugar. Processors did somersaults after realizing the stuff also gave products a boost in flavor and texture, along with a supernatural shelf life. Soft drinks, prepared foods, vending machines -- and our overall access to cheap calories -- would never be the same.

Earl Butz, selected by President Richard Nixon in 1971 to be Secretary of Agriculture, was instrumental in promoting increased corn production. Just a few months before he was cast out of Washington for sharing a crude and racist joke, Butz had ignored the wails of American soybean growers and warnings of health officials. Instead, he negotiated with his counterpart in the government of Malaysia to open the U.S. to massive imports of viscous, orange palm oil.[62]

60: Kelly D. Brownell, Ph.D., and Katherine Battle Horgen, Ph.D. *Food Fight: The Inside Story of the Food Industry, America's Obesity Crisis & What We can Do About It.* New York: McGraw-Hill.
61: Brownell..
62: Greg Critser. *Fat Land: How Americans Became the Fattest People in the World.* Boston: Mariner, 2003.

Never mind that palm oil is a highly saturated fat so similar to beef tallow that critics called it tree lard. It was flavorful, inexpensive and, like HFCS, had a long shelf life.

The new competition from the tropics lowered the price of all oils used in food production and helped solidify our arteries and tolerance for foods that emphasized price over quality. The movement of trains and ships loaded with cheap calories and oils quickly altered the basic mathematics of cooking at home and eating out. Centuries-old dining traditions that placed a premium on flavor, nutrition and presentation were soon replaced by convenience and value, as epitomized by TV dinners and super-sized servings of French fries.

MEGA PORTIONS

The cost of ingredients plummeted. Portions exploded. That 20-ounce plastic bottle of soft drink we leisurely nurse for a couple of hours each morning and/or afternoon provides three times the calories of the 6½-ounce "classic" bottle that was considered refreshing, not bloating, in the days before corn syrup supplanted sugar. The large, 16-ounce fountain Coke once considered a splurge of a purchase when stopping for gasoline now looks like a shot glass beside its successor, the 64-ounce Mega Super Gulp. Today's large order of French fries from McDonald's equals three portions of its original 2-ounce serving, circa 1955. And try finding a 1-ounce hamburger -- typical two generations ago -- at a restaurant that doesn't expect you to put four or more "sliders" on your plate.

Upscale restaurants are likewise expanding portions and offering all-you-can-eat specials to get you through the doors. Bless their generosity, providing you with unlimited plates of pasta or breaded shrimp the size of krill. How can they afford it? Think about that when you order another $3 coffee, $5 beer or $7 slice of cheesecake -- all included on the menu to offset price-shaving elsewhere.

Value-priced meals could be a value if we knew when to quit, but study after study has shown that humans, like rats, will eat more -- as much as 70 percent more — when served larger amounts of food. Food offered in larger packages is rarely broccoli. They're higher-calorie foods which are delectable and easily eaten in large quantities. We tell ourselves we will compensate by eating less the rest of the day, or tomorrow. But we seldom make such adjustments, and studies have shown this, too.

Other changes in society, especially the shift of homemakers moving into paid employment, have turned the occasional meal out into an almost-daily routine for families everywhere. Between 1970 and 2012, the percentage of food dollars spent on food prepared away from home increased from 25.9 percent, to 43.1 percent. Meals at home, meanwhile, are barely homemade. Prepared, frozen breakfasts and dinners tend to also be rich in fats, salt, carbohydrates and sweeteners. They slide easily from freezer to microwave and from lips to hips.

Traditional family meal times are increasingly less distinct, their boundaries blurred by nearly constant snacking in the car, at school, at work, at home, before dinner, after dinner, even at the gym. Restaurant owners have long known that customers eat more when the dining room is kept cool. Now that air-conditioning is pervasive in homes, it's equally comfortable to keep stoking the calories all summer long. And how about those sprawling new houses where kitchens are more than double the size of your grandmother's? Now there is space in the kitchen for larger pantries, a couch or stools for watching TV and, of course, all-day snacking.

LOW-INCOME, HIGH-CALORIE

While all of western civilization has experienced a climate change in food environment, some segments of society have to weather additional hardships. "We think of obesity as being predicted by genetics. Believe me, it is also predicted by incomes and zip codes," says Dr. Adam Drewnowski, a University of Washington (Seattle) nutrition scientist. [63]

The daily cost of special diets low in fats and rich in proteins can easily be double what an average-income person would spend on food. At the same time, the lowest-income families routinely pay more for all types of fresh fruits, vegetables, fish and lean meats — if they're available at all in their neighborhoods. Even after allowing for differences in income, childhood obesity is more common among families in neighborhoods where fresh fruits and vegetables are relatively expensive, the U.S. Department of Agriculture has reported.

Another study, by Tufts University, indicates the "thrifty gene" is highly evident among low-income women for whom access to food is uncertain or inconsistent. Women in food-insecure households were more likely to be obese

63: Craig Degginger. "USDA Study to Address Obesity and Poverty." University of Washington Office of News and Information. June 22, 2004.

and to gain at least 10 pounds in one year, compared to women in fully food-secure households. Researchers hypothesized that when money was tight, the women ate cheaper, high-calorie foods; and when money wasn't so tight, overindulged in traditional comfort foods.[64]

Those among us who are fortunate enough to choose between rib eye or rock lobster or to pay for groceries and fine dining with an American Express card need not succumb to smugness. Yes, obesity has been more prevalent among the poor for decades, but the environment and culture of the middle and upper classes is quickly closing the gap.

A study by the University of Iowa College of Public Health compared waistlines and income, adjusted for inflation. The findings: In the early 1970s, among Americans making less than $25,000 annually, the percentage of obese persons was already high — 22.5 percent. By 2002, the percentage was up to 32.5 percent. But that was a relatively small jump compared to higher income groups. Among those earning $25,000 to $39,999, obesity rates nearly doubled, from 16.1 percent to 31.3 percent. In the income range of $40,000 to $60,000, obesity rates also jumped, from 14.5 percent to 30.3 percent. And among those making more than $60,000 a year, obesity rates nearly tripled, from 9.7 percent to 26.8 percent.[65]

For most of the population today, food is almost an incidental expense, like soap and underwear. Even when Americans and Europeans were first enjoying the prosperity that followed World War II, food claimed only a fifth of disposable income. Today, it is only a tenth, and half of that includes the entertainment value of eating out.

Yup, we've got it good in the neighborhood. Very good. Too good.

NO SWEAT. NOT MUCH, ANYWAY.

The corporations selling high-calorie foods like to blame their customers for enjoying their products to excess without taking on additional exercise to balance the metabolic scales. It's the old "Don't do the crime if you can't do the time" axiom combined with a newer mantra: "calories in = calories out"

64: "Inconsistent Access to Food in Low-Income Households May Contribute to Weight Gain." News release. Tufts University Health Sciences. May 23, 2006.
65: "Obesity No Longer the Domain of the Poor." News-medical.net. May 2, 2005.

But what if exercise doesn't really contribute to weight loss? I know! Blasphemy! But we will sort that out later..

What is true is about the obesogenic environment is that many of the daily routines at home and at work are no longer accomplished by human muscle power. Instead, we spend a few bucks for the gasoline and electricity that powers toothbrushes, dishwashers, garage doors, leaf blowers, SUVs, car windows, elevators and computers.

The path to a better job is still a better education, but usually that ladder leads to a desk job. Even those in more active professions such as sales, nursing, or law enforcement must spend more hours each week seated in front of a computer. And it shows. An Australian study found that men who sit at their desks six hours or more a day are nearly twice as likely to be overweight compared to those who sit for less than 45 minutes a day.

A fair number of desk jockeys ride their Mustangs over to the health club twice a week for a workout sufficient to partly offset a steak dinner or pint of Cherry Garcia. However, the dominant tendency among those whose jobs are physically demanding is to plop hard in an easy chair at every opportunity.

Among children and young adults in all income groups, there is ample evidence that long hours spent in front of a television are more conducive to snacking and weight-gain than hours spent shooting hoops or riding a bike. Computers and video games have only added to the indoor passivity. For a few years, gamers got off their butts to wield a weightless, wireless wand so their video game persona could swing an imaginary golf club, tennis racquet, or broad axe. It was good that mortals had to break a sweat to decapitate a platoon of shuffling zombies. But that got old, too.

Games for motion sensors have fizzled. Kids now are happy to slice flying apples with a single thumb, playing on Mom's smartphone, or their own computer tablet. Older gamers choose a soft throne and settle in for hours of button-mashing.

Neighborhoods matter, too, especially in residential areas perceived to be dangerous. Mothers there breathe easier just knowing their children are safely chillin' by the tube and popping microwaved pizza rolls. Safer, yes. But the mothers who fear their own neighborhoods are also more likely to be obese.

For children, at least, the demise of street ball and after-school playground games should have been offset by more in-school physical education and team sports offerings, especially for girls. Such was the intent of U.S. lawmakers when they passed Title IX of the Education Amendments of 1972, ostensibly opening all school activities to all students, regardless of gender. To the extent they could afford it, public schools began adding staff, locker rooms and practice fields. The benefits of the initiative can be seen today in the widespread success of women's soccer and basketball programs at the high school, collegiate and professional levels.

But budget-strapped school districts, increasingly under pressure to raise academic test scores in the 1980s, 1990s and 2000s, were simultaneously following the path of least resistance, steadily reducing -- then eliminating -- the most basic in-school P.E. programs. Some of the more affluent kids took advantage of the private gyms, swim clubs and after-school soccer leagues that blossomed in the 'burbs. The poor, as usual, were left to absorb the full brunt of budget cuts. All the while, suburban sprawl was making its own unique contribution to the fat-friendly environment. One recent study found the number of trips taken on foot has dropped by 42 percent in two decades. Duh. That would be because "You can't get there from here" -- at least not on foot. Billions of dollars in road construction have linked every Podunk village and farm to every city, shopping center and parking lot, but rarely have included sidewalks, bike paths and crosswalks that provide safe access for children and fitness-minded adults. Unless pressed by local planning and zoning boards, developers of new neighborhoods will continue to skimp on sidewalks, leaving the occasional jogger and skateboarder to share residential streets with the bloated SUVs headed for the nearest convenience stores and burger joints.

GOING VIRAL

Meanwhile, we're learning that many of the antihistamines, antidepressants, and vitamins that provide minor miracles for physical and mental health also contribute to weight gain. And more people are managing to quit smoking, only to be rewarded with extra pounds. Women are waiting longer to have children — and will have heavier babies. Fashionably baggy clothes provide comfortable room to grow — so we fill the available space. Fat people learn to love themselves and each other — then settle down and raise fat children.

Is it something in the air? In the water? Scientists are taking a closer look at a human adenovirus that causes obesity in chickens. One study found that about 30 percent of a group of obese humans examined had antibodies suggesting they may have been exposed to the virus. This raises two interesting questions: Is there a human obesity virus? Is it contagious?

Well, yes, obesity can spread to friends and family members, although the contagion is a social, not viral, phenomenon, according to a headline-grabbing study released by Harvard. [66] Investigators found that as obese individuals become more accepting of their body size, their sensibility spreads, especially to spouses, same-sex siblings and same-sex friends. There's a logical underpinning to the study's finding that such attitudes can be transmitted more readily to the friend of a friend than to a casual neighbor.

However, it is very troubling to think that anyone already harboring prejudice against fat people will use this newest research as an excuse to distance themselves from certain family, friends, or even strangers for fear of "catching" obesity. And you know some will.

If only the creative forces of capitalism could be harnessed to transmit an epidemic of education, understanding, and acceptance with the same blunt force now applied to selling both diet pills and double cheeseburgers to you, your friends and family.

66: Nicholas A. Christakis, M.D., Ph.D, M.P.H. and James H. Fowler, Ph.D. "The Spread of Obesity in a Large Social Network Over 32 Years." *The New England Journal of Medicine.* 357 (2007) : 370-379.

06

EATING, DISORDERED

My mother's mother made great pies with rhubarb culled from a small backyard garden flecked with short rows of greens, beans, and tomatoes. Even as an aging widow, she was careful to prepare sensible meals — usually two vegetables, a lean meat, some bread and sliced peaches for dessert. "I don't live to eat," she once told me, borrowing from Benjamin Franklin to describe her routine. "I eat to live."

Who knows how long she would have lived if a broken hip hadn't limited her ability to move freely? After a few weeks in a rest home, she passed away comfortably. She was 100 years old.

As a school teacher in a small Indiana town, my grandmother in her long life certainly never matched the glamour experienced by Ana Carolina Reston. A rising star in the fashion catwalks of Paris and Milan, the hazel-eyed beauty from Brazil also enjoyed apples and tomatoes — but little else -- in the weeks before she died of kidney failure and collateral infections. At a height of 5 feet 8 inches, Reston weighed 88 pounds. The body mass was typical of a 12-year-old girl's, but she was 21.

In less than a year, Reston had gone from being the featured face and figure in advertising for Armani and Versace to a sorrowful poster child for the self-starvation disease called anorexia nervosa.

It's been 35 years since the 1983 death of singer Karen Carpenter at age 32 first jabbed the eating disorder into popular consciousness. And still, millions of adults and adolescents -- mostly women -- are struggling daily with a morbid fear of fat that stubbornly ignores the primordial link between food and life.

Tens of millions of poor in third-world nations still go hungry the old-fashioned way. They could not comprehend the stylishly hungry who are beaten down by an environment where cheap calories and all-you-can-eat buffets are promoted year-round alongside pitches for skin-tight clothing and 10-day diet plans.

EATING DISORDERS

These powerful, contradictory messages have created a serious and widespread psychosis. Some 24 million American men and women of all ages suffer from an eating disorder --usually anorexia, bulimia, or binge eating. Researchers and treatment specialists say the conditions arise from a combination of factors — not only psychological and sociological, but genetic and neurobiological. As a clinical diagnosis, anorexia is characterized by low body weight and grossly distorted body image. Typically, anorexics resort to any measure short of amputation to shed pounds. Tactics include voluntary starvation and diet pills to restrict caloric intake, followed by vomiting, excessive exercise and diuretic drugs to purge the few calories that are allowed entry.

In addition to perhaps 3.6 million anorexics, the U.S. is home to at least 6 million others — 4.5 million women and 1.5 million men -- classified with bulimia nervosa. Unlike anorexics who are more "successful" in avoiding calories altogether, bulimics may gorge themselves, then attempt to reassert self-control via self-induced vomiting, use of laxatives and water pills, excessive exercise, or fasting. Throughout Canada, Great Britain, Europe, Australia and other Westernized regions of the world, eating disorders (like obesity rates) are increasing to similar and alarming levels. Millions upon millions of individuals otherwise blessed with food to eat now see themselves as fat and disgusting and set a perilous course to become thin and miserable.

Eating disorders have the highest mortality rate of any mental illness.

Even so, fatality estimates may be deceptively low, given that cause-of-death data may not include lives ended by heart attack, organ failure, drug and alcohol abuse or suicide, all rooted in dangerous eating habits.

For survivors of anorexia nervosa, the toll of continued malnutrition includes headaches, constipation, dry lips, creaking joints, sunken eyes, gum disease, pallid complexion, dizziness, and even a growth of the fine lanugo body hair otherwise associated only with fetuses. More severe physical symptoms include abnormalities in the body's mineral and electrolyte levels, endocrine disorders which disrupt menstruation, a slowed heart rate and low blood pressure, tears in the stomach and esophagus, chest pains, and damage to the kidneys, liver and heart. To those effects, add depression, low self-esteem, shame, guilt, mood swings, and a distancing from family and friends.[67]

Those who choose to binge and purge may escape the worst symptoms of starvation, largely because purging doesn't actually work very well for weight loss. Laxatives and diuretics remove mostly water. And half or more of the calories consumed in a binge are absorbed before a vomit intervention is attempted. At best, the bulimic is left with a soul scarred with shame, guilt, and depression. But frequent purging also exposes the body to symptoms of starvation and increases the risk of dehydration, laxative dependence, heart failure, kidney disease and inflammation or even rupture of the esophagus. Just as it is with anorexia nervosa, the worst case is an ugly finish for an eating disorder rooted in an unrealistic quest for beauty.

ADOLESCENT OVERLOAD

Although women are much more likely than men to suffer from eating disorders, the impact is widespread, cutting across boundaries of age, race, and income. The ratio of women to men is about 10 to 1 among older anorexics, but boys may number as much as 30 percent in the youngest age groups, according to the National Association of Anorexia Nervosa and Associated Disorders.

About 86 percent of occurrences appear by the age of 20. Onset occurs between ages 16 and 20 in 43 percent of self-reported cases; 33 percent reported onset between ages 11 and 15; and, most unsettling, 10 percent of those affected are struggling with weight and self-esteem issues before their eleventh birthday.

Expect these numbers continue to grow along with the public's relentless exposure to cultural and media emphasis on fashion and leanness. According to

---

67: National Association of Anorexia and Associated Disorders, *www.anad.org.*.

a survey of 15 years of research by the National Eating Disorders Association:[68]

- An estimated 60 percent of white middle school girls read at least one fashion magazine regularly. Compared to men's magazines, women's magazines have 10.5 times more advertisements and articles promoting weight loss.

- A study of one teen adolescent magazine over two decades found that in articles about fitness or exercise plans, 74 percent cited "to become more attractive" as a reason to start exercising and 51 percent emphasized the need to lose weight or burn calories.

- Girls who diet frequently are 12 times as likely to binge as girls who don't diet.

- More than half of teenage girls and nearly a third of teenage boys use unhealthy weight control behaviors such as fasting, skipping meals, smoking cigarettes, vomiting and taking laxatives.

It's no surprise that girls bear the brunt of cultural attacks on self-esteem. Solidifying the connection, a task force of the American Psychological Association found evidence that the proliferation of sexualized images of girls and young women in advertising, merchandising, and media is harmful to girls' self-image and healthy development.

Many Americans were shocked in 1996 at first seeing pictures of six-year-old murder victim JonBenet Ramsey with the coiffed curls and bright red lipstick she wore for glamorous photo shoots. Ramsey's mother had frequently entered her in the kind of "Little Miss" pageants that have long been a staple of small town celebrations and county fairs. An innocent six-year-old may be able to enjoy the pageantry as a glitzy display of make-believe. But the same element of fantasy can be lost on a 12-year-old girl who uneasily compares her new curves to those of her classmates while avoiding the glares and teasing of the boys. (Boys, I've heard, can be real jerks.)

Adolescents must also compare themselves to the sexually charged images seen on television and in magazines, reinforced by the titillating lyrics and videos

---

68: "Statistics: Eating Disorders and their Precursors," National Eating Disorders Association, *www. nationaleatingdisorders.org.*

for rock, rap and country music. It's not a fair contest. "The consequences of the sexualization of girls in media today are very real and are likely to be a negative influence on girls' healthy development," says Eileen L. Zurbriggen, Ph.D, chair of the psychology task force. Their study linked sexualization and objectification with three of the most common mental health problems diagnosed in girls and women — depression, low self-esteem and eating disorders.[69]

The physical and emotional tremors of puberty and adolescence are something few adults would want to experience again. Yet maturity is no protection against the midlife events that can trigger anorexia or bulimia. About one in 10 patients seeking treatment for eating disorders is over 40. "They've experienced the divorce, the death of a parent or both parents, a traumatic illness like breast cancer, children leaving home," says Dr. Ed Cumella, an eating disorders specialist in Arizona. "Any woman with low self-esteem who has gone through that kind of life stressor is at risk."[70]

FOOD ADDICTIONS AND BINGEING

Within the overweight and obese population, unrestrained eating and outright bingeing are the more common eating disorders. Scenarios range from the ritualistic ingestion of a favorite soft drink, candy bar or pint of ice cream to daylong grazing or, at its most extreme, an uncontrollable gorging, usually conducted in secret and always followed by feelings of misery and guilt.

William Leith, a British journalist who has battled bingeing since childhood, has described the beginning of his recurring episodes in chilling terms:

"When it happens, when the terrible thing happens, it arrives quietly, surreptitiously, like the sort of storm that kills sailors when they can't see it coming. One minute you're fine, and then, click: you're in a different world . . . You have fallen down a hole."[71]

Although binge eating wasn't formally classified by the American Psychiatric Association as a specific eating disorder until 2013, experts generally

69: "Sexualization of Girls is Linked to Common Mental Health Problems in Girls and Women: Eating Disorders," *American Psychological Association* (APA) news release via Newswise, © 2007.
70: "Anorexia Also Strikes Middle-Aged Women," *ABC News*, October 15, 2005, ©2005 ABC News Internet Ventures.
71: William Leith. *Confessions of a Food Addict.* New York: Gotham Books, 2005.

agreed that two out-of-control binges a week was enough to be considered a serious problem warranting medical intervention.

Although obesity is not consistent evidence of binge eating, binge eaters are frequently overweight and at further risk of high blood pressure, heart disease and diabetes -- all conditions requiring medical attention. But researchers say bingeing, like anorexia and bulimia, is usually associated with more deep-seated problems.[72]

Other surveys have shown that about half of those with bulimia suffered from major depression or phobias and a third were substance abusers. One study concluded that more than 94 percent of people with bulimia, 56 percent of those with anorexia and 79 percent of those with binge-eating disorder had at least one other psychiatric diagnosis.[73]

Less clear is which comes first — the depression or the eating disorder. Certainly, one can feed the other.

AND STILL MORE EATING DISORDERS

Meanwhile, other researchers are attaching names to a new group of eating disorders still formally classified as NOS, or "not otherwise specified" in the official diagnostic manual of the American Psychiatric Association. Formal classifications aren't just academic. They open the door to drug treatments that are promoted by drug makers and resisted by insurance companies, each because of their strong financial interests.

Two such disorders fall on the health fanatic side of the spectrum. While most of us don't get enough exercise, a few others, especially teens and athletes, have migrated to compulsive, excessive, and harmful amounts of physical activity. Used as device for weight control, the condition has been named *anorexia athletica,* or sport anorexia. Other studies have found a high frequency of disordered eating among competitive athletes, especially among women and in sports which put a premium on endurance (such as distance running),

72: "Study Tracks Prevalence of Eating Disorders," *National Institute of Mental Health,* Science Update, February 9, 2007. The study referenced represented a survey or more than 2,980 men and women and was conducted by researchers from Harvard University and McLean Hospital in Belmont, Mass. See: "The Prevalence and Correlates of Eating Disorders in the National Comorbidity Survey Replication," *Biological Psychiatry* 2007; 61:348-358).
73: Nicholas Bakalar . "Survey Puts New Focus on Binge Eating as a Diagnosis." *The New York Times,* February 13, 2007.

aesthetics (gymnastics), or classification by weight (wrestling). In one survey, a fourth of the athletes reported bingeing at least once a week. Abuse of laxatives or enemas was common. And researchers are now paying more attention to a subgroup of finicky eaters who have taken their fear or contempt for heavily processed foods to an extreme by limiting themselves to a few morsels of "righteous" foods. They may attach a near-spiritual belief in the power of tofu and bean sprouts, even to the point of emaciation. This one has been named *orthorexia nervosa*.

Researchers also are beginning to find connections between eating disorders and an individual's brain chemistry, metabolism, and genetic history. Studies of families have found that individuals with a mother or sister who has suffered from anorexia are 12 more times likely to adopt the disorder. With bulimia in particular, investigators have concluded that genes on three different chromosomes significantly affect risk levels. The genes were linked to six core traits which influence eating disorders: obsessiveness or perfectionism, anxiety, concern over mistakes, lifetime BMI, age at first menstruation and, of course, food-related obsessions.[74]

This much is certain. Those who are still in hiding with the physical and mental burden of an eating disorder need to get their butts out of the bathroom and their heads out of the refrigerator and march into the offices of a health professional. Political Correctness has been set aside here for the greater good of reaching those in denial. If that applies to you, first see a medical professional, *then* write me a nasty letter if you're still offended.

Effective treatments are available for those who will just seek it out. Dieting is *not* the answer, at least not until more serious problems are addressed. Instead, physicians and counselors may recommend any of several treatment methods already found to be highly effective. Cognitive-behavioral therapy teaches people how to change their unhealthy eating habits and be better prepared to deal with stressful situations. Interpersonal psychotherapy helps people look at their relationships with friends and family and make changes in problem areas.

Drug therapy, such as antidepressants, may be helpful for some people, but anyone for whom a drug is recommended should insist on the physician's full

---

74: "Researchers Identify Core Traits Strongly Linked to Eating Disorders." News release, University of North Carolina at Chapel Hill School of Medicine, September 9, 2005.

disclosure of the potential risks and side effects, followed up by more research and another round of talks with the doctor. Then, if your doctor determines a prescription is necessary or worth trying, ask about starting with the smallest appropriate dosage. I'm still not a doctor, but I can prescribe ample research for all patients and candid communication with all medical providers.

Millions of others — possibly you -- are not in danger or denial but still worried about benign food addictions. Talk about it with friends and family or hook up with some imperfect strangers through an established, not-for-profit support group such as Take Off Pounds Sensibly (TOPS) or Overeaters Anonymous. You may need to visit several groups. Some locals are stridently fussy about weigh-ins and forbidden foods. If you find a chapter that ends their meetings with chicken wings and buttermilk pie, let me know. You know, just for research purposes.

07

DIETING, DISORDERED

There is one more major eating disorder awaiting a formal entry in diagnostic manuals, even though it's the most obvious and prevalent, affecting as many as 115 million Americans, or one in three adults. Symptoms include:

- Fear of maintaining a normal body weight for age and height.

- Intense fear of gaining weight, or becoming fat.

- Undue influence of body weight or shape on self-image.

- Engaging in compulsive eating rituals with obsessive categorization of individual foods as good or bad.

All these symptoms have been applied to anorexia nervosa. But take another look. Don't most of these describe a typical weight-loss dieter? Do they describe you? Probably, if you are one of the 70 million Americans dieting to lose weight or the 45 million struggling to maintain an unnatural weight.

Especially for women, the pressure to maintain an unnatural thinness has long percolated through fashion. Unhappily, the glamorized "ideal" weight has dropped almost continuously since the arrival of the Gibson Girl in the 1890s and the even-thinner flappers of the 1920s. Today, the willowy shadows of young models, singers and actresses keep the pressure on peers and fans to believe less is always more.

Sports Illustrated broke with its spindly tradition in 2016 by putting model Ashley Graham on the cover of its annual swimsuit edition. At size 14 and 166 pounds, Graham was quite close to the size of the average American woman. Yet, the magazine scored more free publicity than usual because Graham is considered plus-size in the fantasy world of film and fashion.

One lifestyle magazine for teens surveyed its readers and found that 30 percent would rather be thin than healthy. Two-thirds of young women in another survey said compared to being fat, it's better to be mean or stupid[75] -- a good indication that two-thirds of the survey group is already being fat-shamed, shaming others, or is shamefully self-absorbed. More forgivingly, we could say an uninformed majority is suffering from culturally-induced eating disorders.

If every dieter who failed gave up after the first attempt, there would be only a third as many dieters. But dieters try, and try again, and try once more, even though 95 percent are destined to continue failing.

You'll find a more positive spin on the success of weight-loss dieting if you look at the materials cited by the companies marketing diet programs and supplies, and even by some government and university studies that promote such diets. What those studies usually have in common is a short follow-up period, often a year or less, or an over-reliance on self-reporting by survey subjects who underestimate their current weights.

Somebody should thoroughly study the success of dieters over a period of two to five years. Somebody did! A team of psychologists at the University of California Los Angeles conducted their own rigorous analysis of 31 different long-term weight-loss studies. You'll like only one of their findings — that it's easy to initially lose 5 to 10 percent of your weight on any number of diet plans.

"But then the weight comes right back," said Traci Mann, then a UCLA associate professor of psychology and lead author of the study. "We found that the majority of people regained all the weight, *plus more*. Sustained weight loss was found only in a small minority of participants."[76]

75: Courtney E. Martin. "One Big Fat Lie," an article posted at *www.alternet.org*, March 2, 2006 and adapted from her book, *Perfect Girls, Starving Daughters: The Frightening New Normalcy of Hating Your Body*, published by Free Press, April 17, 2007.

76: "Dieting Does Not Work, Researchers Report." University of California, Los Angeles news release as reported by www.sciencedaily.com. April 5, 2007.

The study found that within five years at least one-third and as many as two-thirds of people on diets *put on more pounds than they lose*

Another key finding also goes without celebration. Several of the 31 studies indicated that dieting is actually a consistent predictor of future weight gain, not only for obese people, but for those who start at a moderate weight.

Mann, now teaching psychology at the University of Minnesota, has continued her research and is all the more convinced that dieters are too hard on themselves. Diets fail because of the physical and psychological changes brought on by calorie-cutting, she says. Neurologically, dieters are rewiring themselves so that the very foods they are trying to cut out become even more tempting. At the same time, the hormones which drive hunger and control satiety shift out of balance, pushing the dieter to crave the missing calories.

Third, and most powerfully, the dieter's metabolism slows down. "Your body uses calories in the most efficient way possible. . .which would be a good thing if you're starving to death," Mann says. "When your body finds a way to run itself on fewer calories there tends to be more left over, and those get stored as fat, which is exactly what you don't want to happen."[77]

With all that physiology working to maintain a body's natural weight range, Mann says she hates for dieters to blame themselves. Willpower is extremely useful in many areas of life, such as improving test scores, she says, "but when it comes to eating, it's just not the problem. It's not the fix."[78]

DANGER: DIETING AHEAD

So, for most people, dieting to *lose* weight is ultimately the same as charting a twisted, frustrating and exhausting route to *gain* weight. Reality check: Wouldn't it be a lot easier to enjoy your favorite foods in moderation, get a little more exercise and slowly add a few pounds? Easier by a mile, I'd say, and according to 70 years of medical research, healthier by two miles.

Physiologist Ancel Keys became famous, first of all, for developing the compact packages of food carried into combat in World War II. He's the K in

---

77: Roberto A. Ferdman. "Why Diets Don't Actually Work, According to a Researcher Who Has Studied Them For Decades." *Washingtonpost.com*. May 4, 2015.

78: Ferdman.

K-rations. They couldn't call them TV dinners back then because there was no TV. Also, the original MREs (meals, ready to eat) came with some toilet paper and four cigarettes. Later, Keys did pioneering research on the relationship between blood cholesterol and heart disease. Later, he championed the Mediterranean style diet. He lived to be 100, which is a good way to advocate from beyond the grave.

The same researcher was also famous for his 1944 study of 36 conscientious objectors to military service who were confined at the University of Minnesota and, with the War Department's permission, placed on semi-starvation diets for 24 weeks. Their carefully controlled rations were low in calories, but included adequate amounts of protein, vitamins and minerals. During the dieting phase, the men lost weight rapidly and soon became irritable, quarrelsome, lethargic and depressed. Can you relate? In fact, two of the volunteers suffered complete emotional breakdowns and a third chopped off the end of his finger, evidently hoping to get three squares a day while in the infirmary. (If the others fought over who would eat the severed digit, it was not reported.)

Some fifteen weeks after the experiment ended with a much-anticipated banquet, the men were returning to their old personalities but still obsessed with food. Although allowed to eat whatever they wished, the men reported feeling near-constant hunger for some nine months, until recovering their original amounts of body fat and muscle -- and then some.

"In fact six of the men ended up with an average of 9 ½ pounds more body fat than they had before entering what became, in effect, the first 'yo-yo' dieting experiment," physiologist Glenn A. Gaesser wrote in *Big Fat Lies*, his ahead-of-its-time book, published in 1996.[79] Now a professor and specialist in exercise science at Arizona State University, Gaesser was one of a handful of writers with sound academic credentials to challenge entrenched theories about weight and health. He did it by connecting the dots using decades of research which had been marginalized for being out of sync with Conventional Wisdom.

Some of the most powerful information came from a study too horrible to construct. For 900 days, beginning in October 1941, the German siege of Leningrad (now St. Petersburg, Russia) trapped residents in a near-starvation

---

79: Glenn A Gaesser, Ph.D. *Big Fat Lies: The Truth About Your Weight and Your Health.* Fawcett Columbine. New York. 1996.

diet. More than a million died. It's what happened after the siege was lifted that was surprising. A study of 10,000 Leningraders, male and female, before and after, showed that in addition to regaining lost weight, the incidents of high blood pressure among survivors had doubled or quadrupled, depending on their ages. Pre-siege, autopsies revealed less than six percent had vascular damage resulting from hypertension. More than a year after food supplies returned to normal, vascular disease was evident in more than half of autopsies. The consistencies between the Leningrad siege and the Minnesota experiment impressed Keys and his associates enough to formally voice, in 1948, "the possibility that such a patient may be worse off, when he modifies or abandons his dietary restrictions, than he was *before* the treatment was instituted."[80]

Short version: Yo-yo dieting is worse than no yo at all.

11 HOURS OF LIFE

Gaesser, then an associate professor of exercise physiology at the University of Virginia, reviewed 17 studies conducted between 1983 and 1993. He found that all but two of them showed that weight loss *increased* the risk of premature death by up to 260 percent. "And of the two studies in the minority, one showed an 11-hour increase in longevity per pound of weight lost — not exactly a ringing endorsement!" [81] Nope. To gain a year of life at that rate, one would have to lose 796 pounds.

So that's just some of the unconventional wisdom that's been blipping slightly beyond mainstream media's radar for 70 years or more. More recent studies have continued to show the dangers of extreme or repetitive weight loss, especially for those without serious medical problems. Men and women whose weight cycled often or greatly over a period of many years had a significantly higher risk of death than who were steadily overweight, according to a large-scale U.S. study published in 1998. A 25-year study of 3,000 people in Finland also concluded that overweight people who dieted to reach a healthier weight were more likely to die younger than those who remained fat. [82] In particular, healthy overweight or obese who tried to lose weight and succeeded over a

---

80: Gaesser.
81: Gaesser.
82: Abigail Wild. "Can Diets Cut Your Life Short?" *The Herald* (London) June 30, 2005.
Thorkild Sorensen, and others. "Intention to Lose Weight, Weight Changes, and 18-y Mortality in Over-
    weight Individuals Without Co-Morbidities." PLoS Med 2(6) (2005): e171

six-year period had almost double the risk of dying during the next 18 years, compared with subjects who did not try to lose weight and whose weight remained stable.[83]

Those researchers and other nutritionists say that extreme weight loss breaks down important protein mass in the body compared to more moderate calorie-cutting with exercise, which removes a higher percentage of fat. Still, other studies have linked weight-cycling with increased risk for destroying heart tissue, stroke, diabetes and suppressed immune function. And a study of more than 51,000 men in the U.S. found the risk of gallstone disease was 40 percent higher in men who had lost and regained 20 pounds at least once.[84]

All this research and more is what led Mann and her UCLA associates to reach a conclusion that may anger some dieters and the diet industry while siding with taxpayers in general. "We are recommending that Medicare should not fund weight-loss programs as a treatment for obesity," Mann said. "The benefits of dieting are too small and the potential harm is too large for dieting to be recommended as a safe, effective treatment for obesity."[85]

(*RESULTS NOT TYPICAL)

Even without federal subsidies, weight loss remains a strong and healthy segment of the U.S. economy. One relatively conservative estimate is that weight-loss services alone churn $2.4 billion in sales annually. Oh, but there's more. Lots more. Add to that the cost of medical and commercial weight-loss programs, prescription and over-the-counter weight-loss pills, meal replacements, low-calorie dinner entrees, bariatric surgeries, artificial sweeteners, diet soft drinks, diet books and exercise videos. Now we're talking about a $60 billion chunk of the economy, equal to all new U.S. credit card debt in 2015.

Spending in the segments has been changing somewhat: for example, less spending on diet drinks and more on sugary "hydration" blends, marketed as blue, green, yellow, or red liquids, for no apparent reason. Totals sales, however, have been declining 3 or 4 percent annually.

83: "Can Losing Weight Be Unhealthy?" *myDNA News*, posted online January 28, 2005.
84: Judith Groch. "Gallstone Disease in Men Built on Weight Cycling." *www.medpagetoday.com*, November 27, 2006.
85: "Dieting Does Not Work, UCLA Researchers Report," news release from University of California – Los Angeles, April 3, 2007.

Anyone who has tried on their own and failed to keep weight off is an easy target for the commercial weight-loss programs. Advertising typically features photos and testimonials from attractive customers (a.k.a. professional models) who say they've lost 30, 50 or a 100 pounds or more just by "following the plan." Such headlines are inevitably followed by the most powerful punctuation mark in all of advertising — the asterisk, as in "*Results not typical. Individual results may vary." At least you can pause to read the fine print in a magazine advertisement. Good luck deciphering more than a few words in the disclaimers on television advertisements. They're hidden somewhere in that full screen of squished legalese visible for maybe three seconds of airtime.

So what is it the diet marketers are so eager not to tell you? Probably it's that their success rates — if they have kept any data at all — are generally no better than what you can achieve on your own. Even if you pay attention to the disclaimers, the implication is that if you don't get good results, the fault is yours, not theirs.

Aware that many physicians would rather refer overweight patients to a commercial plan than provide the necessary counseling and motivation themselves, a team of researchers at the University of Pennsylvania attempted to evaluate and compare the methods, costs, and effectiveness of the most popular weight-loss programs.[86]

They scoured the companies' websites and reviewed 108 related studies, but found only 10 deemed comprehensive enough to be valid. And while some programs were eager to tout their typical results after a period of three to six months, only Weight Watchers could produce legitimate randomized trials sustained for at least two years. Weight Watchers reported weight loss of 5.3 percent after six months, with customers typically regaining all but 3.2 percent of their starting weight after two years. The study's authors estimated the cost of the Weight Watchers plan at $841* for two years — considerably less than most other plans compared, which generally included professional medical counseling and/or the cost of replacement meals. But let's assume, for the sake

---

86: Tsai, Adam Gilden, MD, and Thomas A. Wadden, PhD. "Systematic Review: An Evaluation of Major Commercial Weight Loss Programs in the United States." *Annals of Internal Medicine.* January 2005. The commercial plans compared were Weight Watchers, Jenny Craig, L.A. Weight Loss, Health Management Resources, OPTIFAST, Medifast/Take Shape for Life, eDiets.com. Two non-profit, self-help programs, Take Off Pounds Sensibly (TOPS) and Overeaters Anonymous, were also compared where relevant.

of easy math, someone using Weight Watchers started with 200 pounds. Losing 6.4 pounds over two years cost them about $263* per pound lost. (*Here, I've adjusted for inflation, converting the 2004 data to 2015 dollars.)

DREAM FACTORY

Perhaps the key finding of the study was that the weight-loss industry is allowed to operate in such secrecy, particularly with respect to its long-term success rates. Ideally, the U.S. Federal Trade Commission would require the commercial programs to monitor and report their outcomes. But the FTC doesn't have that power, according to Richard Cleland, the FTC's assistant director for advertising practices. In the mid-1990s, the FTC tried unsuccessfully to get the major weight-loss vendors to agree to voluntary guidelines, Cleland told the New York Times.

"In general, the industry has always been opposed to making outcomes disclosures." Their reasons, he said, range from claims that monitoring is too expensive to "even arguing that part of this is selling the dream, and if you know what the truth is, it's harder to sell the dream."[87]

Well, no shite, Sherlock. Think how many opportunists would rather "sell the dream" of a miracle diet pill, cancer cure, or get-rich-quick scheme without regard for the truth. More puzzling is how elected leaders and regulators decide which practices to reign in and which to ignore.

Perhaps diet programs get a pass because their customers have a greater influence on outcomes than the program themselves. In truth, it's possible to lose weight by following any of hundreds of diets and diet plans. But how much weight? And how long before diet fatigue sets in and the weight begins to return?

A separate study by a team at Boston's Tufts-New England Medical Center randomly assigned 40 volunteers to each of four popular diets: Weight Watchers, which stressed calorie control; the Atkins low-carbohydrate plan; the Zone Diet, which emphasizes glycemic loads and nutritional balance; and the low-fat vegetarian plan promoted by Dr. Dean Ornish.

87: Gina Kolata. "Diet and Lose Weight? Scientists Say 'Prove It!'" *The New York Times*, January 4, 2005.

After two months of coaching, each participant was left to fly solo until their big weigh-in at the end of 12 months, whether they stuck with the plan or not. Weight Watchers and the Zone plan had the best stick-with-it rating, with 65 percent still participating for the full year. Participants lost an average of 6.6 pounds and 7.1. pounds, respectively. In the Atkins group, 53 percent stayed with it and weight loss averaged 4.6 pounds. The Ornish group had the highest losses, 7.3 pounds on average, but only half of the group could last a year.[88]

Dr. Thomas Wadden, lead author of the University of Pennsylvania study and director of a weight and eating disorders program there, said he wasn't surprised that diet programs resulted in only modest or temporary weight loss. "I don't blame the diet programs. They're fighting biology," Wadden said. "Even in the best of circumstances, people will regain a third of what they lost in one year and two-thirds in two years, and they may be back to baseline in five years. Weight loss," he cautioned, "is not for the faint-hearted."[89]

Nor is weight loss for amateurs with a poor understanding of basic nutrition. Yet many diet programs, especially those promising the fastest results, rely on nutrition shortcuts and calorie counts that leave your basic body building blocks teetering.

ORGANIZED FAILURE

Not long ago, a former women's wellness counselor for what she called a "popular weight loss company" interrupted the internet's usual weight-loss pity party with a personal and powerful blog post. "An Open Apology to All of My Weight Loss Clients," by Iris Higgins first appeared on her blog site and was quickly re-posted by dozens of major news outlets and shared with thousands more via social media. An insider was revealing the industry's most important secret.

"I'm sorry," Higgins began. Here's an abbreviated, still potent edit of what followed: [90]

88: DeNoon, Daniel. "4 Diets Face Off: Which is the Winner?" *www.WebMD.com*, January 4, 2005. Also, M.Dansinger. *Journal of the American Medical Association*. Jan. 5, 2005.

89: Kolota.

90: Iris Higgins. "An Open Letter to All of My Weight Loss Clients." *www.yourfairyangel.com*, July 27, 2013. Higgins has an M.A. degree in psychology with additional studies in nutrition and a certification in hypnotherapy. A former rugby player, she has authored two guides to gluten-free baking and offers counseling services to women.

"I'm sorry because I put you on a 1200 calorie diet and told you that was healthy. I'm sorry because when you were running five times a week, I encouraged you to switch from a 1200 calorie diet to a 1500 calorie diet, instead of telling you that you should be eating a hell of a lot more than that. I'm sorry because you were breastfeeding and there's no way eating those 1,700 calories a day could have been enough for both you and your baby.

I'm sorry because I made you feel like a failure and so you deliberately left a message after the center had closed, telling me you were quitting. I thought you were awesome and gorgeous, and I'm sorry because I never told you that.

I am sorry because many of you walked in healthy and walked out with disordered eating, disordered body image, and the feeling that you were a "failure." None of you ever failed. Ever. I failed you. The weight loss company failed you. Our society is failing you.

I'm sorry because I get it now. If you're trying to starve your body by eating fewer calories than it needs, of course it's going to fight back.

Just eat food. Eat real food, be active, and live your life. Forget all the diet and weight loss nonsense. It's really just that. Nonsense."

B.S. IN A BOTTLE

Knowing that diets are difficult and diet programs are iffy, perhaps I could interest you in an easy alternative -- a product called McGowan's Reducine. By using it, the maker says, "excess fat is literally dissolved away, leaving the figure slim and properly rounded, giving the lithe grace to the body every man and woman desires." Better yet, Reducine can be applied only to those body areas you want to slenderize, "quickly, surely and permanently." [91]

If you find that tempting, I'd also like to show you some property below the New Orleans flood plain that would be perfect for development.

Reducine was advertised in 1927 in the pages of *True Romances* magazine. It was significant not because it was the only advertised product of its type, but

---

91: "Protecting Consumers From False And Deceptive Advertising Of Weight-Loss." Hearing Before The Subcommittee On Consumer Protection, Product Safety, And Insurance. The Committee On Commerce Science, And Transportation , United States Senate. One Hundred Thirteenth Congress Second Session. June 17, 2014

because the U.S. Federal Trade Commission found its claims ludicrous enough to, for the first time, initiate punitive legal action. Since then, thousands of similar products have appeared on the market and stayed around long enough to snare of new group of suckers. Then they drop from view, only to resurface with a new name and P.O. box number.

Although the names changed often enough to protect the guilty, the advertising methods have remained much the same. Amazingly, in an age when "The Nanny State" seeks to protect us from injury by requiring inane warning labels ("Do not iron while wearing shirt." "Do not hold the wrong end of chainsaw."), deceptive advertisements for weight-loss products continue to proliferate, even in mainstream media.

To be clear, the FDA has primary jurisdiction over prescription drugs and the *labeling* of over-the-counter drugs and dietary supplements, while the FTC has authority over the *advertising* of over-the-counter drug products, devices and dietary supplements.

The last big study of trends in weight-loss advertising by the staff of the Federal Trade Commission compared issues of popular magazines published during the spring of 1992 and the same months of 2001. [92]

"The change in the extent and tenor of weight-loss advertising has been dramatic," the FTC staffers reported. The biggest jump by far — a twelve fold increase -- was in the shilling of dietary supplements.

In addition to the group of glossy magazines, the FTC team collected a total of 300 advertising specimens from a variety of tabloid, newspaper, television and radio advertisements, as well as TV "infomercials," direct mail and the Internet. They found a "virtual fantasy land" of rapturous claims and blurry disclaimers, all delivered without the slightest hint of a wink. Most of the smoke-and-mirrors fell into these categories:

- Consumer testimonials: By far the most common technique, testimonials were featured in 65 percent of the samples. And they weren't describing modest or realistic results. Weight losses cited in 195 testimonials averaged 71 pounds. Only a third of the testimonial

---

92: Richard L. Cleland, and others. "Weight-Loss Advertising: An Analysis of Current Trends." A report by the staff of the Federal Trade Commission, September 2002.

ads included "results not typical" or any disclaimer at all.

- Before-and-after photos: These showed up in 42 percent of advertising samples. Typically, the "before" photo has a grainy, snapshot quality with poor lighting and washed out skin tones. Subjects are seemingly chosen for their poor posture, blank expressions, unkempt hair, baggy clothes or protruding stomachs. "After" photos, not surprisingly, feature flattering studio lighting, a beach-ready body, stylish hair and make-up, perfect posture and a skimpy bathing suit.[93]

Also in common misuse were such bromides as "guaranteed results," "all-natural ingredients," "safe and effective," "no dieting or exercise required," "permanent results," "clinically proven," and "medically approved."

Of course, all of these claims came with little or no documentation or verifiable specifics. My favorites, in terms of sheer chutzpah, were the ones claiming to be so effective that customers should be prepared to reduce use of the miracle pills in the event of "excessive weight loss."

However well-intentioned, the Federal Trade Commission seems to only have enough resources to go after the worst (that is, most successful) offenders.

I hope you were not among the millions who paid $59 (plus shipping and handling -- Can't forget the shipping and handling!) for a one-month supply of a miracle condiment. Just sprinkle a little on your food, the TV, radio and print ads said, and the flavor enhancers would make you feel full faster, eat less and lose weight. The claims generated $364 million in sales in just four years. When the FTC finished its investigation, California-based Sensa Products, LLC, related companies and individuals were fined $46.5 million for their deceptive advertising and unsubstantiated claims.[94]

The FTC's comparison of most weight-loss claims to a "fantasy land" is accurate. Unfortunately, the same is true of the FTC's appeal to the industry to voluntarily limit itself to realistic claims, and for publishers and broadcasters to voluntarily set higher standards for advertisers. When money talks, ethics balk.

93: Cleland.

94: "Sensa and Three Others Marketers of Fad Weight-Loss Products Settle FTC Charges in Crack-down on Deceptive Advertising." www.ftc.gov. January 7, 2014.

Fat and smart consumers will just have to maintain a healthy skepticism about any product or service targeted at the fat and gullible.

08

PILLS AND KILLS

SUPPLEMENTS AND PRESCRIPTION MEDICINES CHASE PROFITS AND DREAMS

I just happen to live in a town -- I assume the only one in the world -- where most grocery stores stock gallon jugs of Worcestershire sauce year-round. It's not that Owensboro, KY was founded by Misters Lea and Perrins, or that we share an addiction to the black gold's secret ingredient (anchovies!).

In our one little slice of Western Kentucky, barbecued mutton is king. It's slow-cooked over a smoldering wood fire during a full summer of church picnics, kicked off by a festival each May that attracts thousands of people. The big racks of mutton, pork and chicken are kitchen-mopped with vats of tangy dip made with Worcestershire, vinegar and other If-we-told-you-we'd-have-to-kill-you ingredients.

Festivals are great for eating because there is so much walking and standing involved. Too bad our regular food culture doesn't require as much physical effort to locate, harvest, and prepare a solid meal. But hunt we shall for a genuine weight-loss miracle in the form of a prescription formula produced by a big pharmaceutical company or some over-the-counter blend packaged and marketed as a "dietary supplement."

Vitamin, mineral, and herbal concentrates and blends, along with other forms of alternative or complementary medicine, are a $37 billion-a-year business in the United States alone. As much as anything, their success demonstrates Americans' dissatisfaction with traditional health care remedies. Largely unproven and unregulated, they promise anything from thinner thighs and thicker hair to relief from arthritis or a reprieve from cancer.

The curatives offer hope, even to users who concede their value may be purely psychological. Buyers "do not appear to care that there is little, if any, evidence that many of the therapies work," as science reporter Benedict Carey wrote in the *New York Times.* "Nor do they seem to mind that alternative therapy practitioners have a fraction of the training mainstream doctors do, or that vitamin and herb makers are as profit-driven as drug makers."[95]

The proliferation of unproven supplements got its biggest boost from none other than the U.S. Congress when it approved a 1994 measure called the Dietary Supplement Health and Education Act. The "Education" part evidently implies that we should educate ourselves, because the chief failure of the act was to excuse supplement sellers from first submitting clinical evidence of their products' safety and effectiveness to the U.S. Food and Drug Administration. Soon after, pharmacy shelves were awash with hundreds of weight-loss products derived from herbs and botanicals, minerals, enzymes, and/or organ tissues.

With a fifth or more of the public actively attempting to lose weight at any given time, it's easy to see how supplements marketed to dieters are so profitable. More than half of that spending is by consumers who mistakenly believe they are buying products which had been scientifically verified as effective and federally approved for safety.[96]

In a nation where so many decry the nanny state and intrusive government regulation, here is a major industry succeeding because of the mistaken belief the feds have given a thumbs up for every product sold for ingestion.

The modern history of medicinal fat-fighting is marked by short-term successes, long-term regrets and more than a few fatalities. Wasn't anyone saying "If it sounds too good to be true . . . "?

95: Benedict Carey. "When Trust in Doctors Erodes, Other Treatments Fill the Void." *The New York Times.* February 3, 2006.
96: Jane E. Brody. "Weight-Loss Drugs: Hoopla and Hype," The New York Times, April 24, 2007.

EPHEDRA

In the mid-1990s, products containing ephedra or its synthetic cousin, phenylpropanolamine (PPA), were selling quickly under various names, including the highly marketed Metabolife, Dexatrim and Acutrim. This occurred as the FDA was warning of potential adverse health effects, especially among persons with high blood pressure, heart disease and diabetes. One 1998 study showed use of PPA was as high as 3.5 percent of all adult women. The same survey also showed that more than a tenth of men and a third of women using prescription weight-loss pills also reported taking ephedra or PPA. [97]

Native Americans and Mormon pioneers are said to have occasionally brewed a tea from ephedra plants, just as the Chinese had done for 5,000 years as a remedy for colds and asthma, but not with the frequency or potency of the tablets being sold by the millions as a shortcut to weight loss. Dosages varied, not only from brand to brand, but from batch to batch. At the same time ephedra was being embraced by dieters, its reputation as a stimulant and "performance enhancer" made it equally popular with night-drivers, students, and athletes.

Regardless of their motivation, all users were subject to any of the same side effects: nervousness, trembling, dehydration, irregular heartbeat, heart attack, stroke — and death. After the FDA proposed stricter labeling in 1997, the supplement makers launched their own "objective" studies and organized a multi-million lobbying campaign. The lobbying effort kept Congress and regulators at bay until 2002 when the U.S. Department of Justice, under pressure from the consumer advocacy group Public Citizen, forced ephedra's top defender, Metabolife, to open up its files. And there they were: reports of 15,000 adverse reactions ranging from insomnia to death, all of which the company had previously withheld from the FDA. Legal challenges followed, as did the deaths of several prominent athletes. It wasn't until February 2007 that the FDA was finally able to enforce a ban on all ephedra products.

Ephedra's chemical cousin, phenylpropanolamine (PPA), enjoyed several years of mainstream acceptance, not just in weight-control concoctions, but as a decongestant in cold formulas sold under such well-known brands as Alka-Seltzer, Tavist-D, Triaminic, Dimetapp, Robitussin, Comtrex and Sine Off.

97: Heidi Michels Blanck, PhD, and others. "Use of Nonprescription Weight Loss Products: Results from a Multistate Survey." *Journal of the American Medical Association.* Vol. 286. August 22, 2001.

Some versions also were recommended for children. As with ephedra, the burden of proof was upon the FDA to show the ingredient was not safe, rather than requiring its makers to prove it was safe before going to market — again because of the 1994 act.

While psychiatrists were linking PPA to diagnoses of acute mania and paranoid schizophrenia, two other studies had confirmed a suspected link between PPA and hemorrhagic stroke in women. Again, the FDA moved slowly. In 2000, it issued a public health advisory and *requested* ("Pretty, pretty, please?") an end to products made with phenylpropanolamine.

An outright ban on the over-the-counter sales would wait another five years, when the emphasis had shifted to preventing its use in the illegal manufacture of dangerous and addictive methamphetamine. Yes, meth.

Nature abhors a vacuum. The physics maxim also applies to the marketing of natural foods and dietary supplements. Even as ephedra and PPA were being pulled from the shelves, supplement makers were introducing new weight-loss capsules containing blends of caffeine and extracts from other herbs, including the newest star in the weight-loss firmament, bitter orange.

Not surprisingly, the ephedra substitutes may pose some of the same cardiovascular risks. The primary constituents of bitter orange extract are similar to pharmaceutical synephrine and have the same capacity to increase heart rate and raise blood pressure, especially when combined with the equivalent of three cups of coffee -- the amount of caffeine actually added to one formula tested. Further study of the long-term effect of the products is needed, the researchers said. Until then, they said, "physicians should caution patients about the use of ephedra-free weight-loss dietary supplements, and monitor blood pressure in those who choose to use these supplements."[98]

HOODIA GORDONII

The 21st Century dawned with a new herbal star on the horizon, one with a name and origin so exotic one would expect King Kong himself to be guarding the plant nursery. I'm speaking of hoodia gordonii, a juicy-leaf, cactus-like plant

---

98: Minerd, Jeff, "Ephedra-Free Supplements Not Necessarily Risk-Free," *www.medpagetoday.com.*, September 12, 2005. The study cited by Christine A. Haller, M.D., and colleagues, appeared in the *American Journal of Medicine*, September 9, 2005.

native only to the Kalahari Desert of southern Africa. The San Bushmen of the Kalahari, deprived as they were of gossip magazines, juice bars, and fitness clubs, never felt a need to quickly shed 10 pounds before bathing suit season. However, generations of the primitive tribesmen have snacked on hoodia to suppress hunger during long hunting trips.

Does it really work? Yes, according to a BBC correspondent who made the pilgrimage to the Kalahari in 2003. And yes, according to a correspondent for CBS TV's "60 Minutes" who made the trip in 2004. The hoodia hoopla spread quickly after that, but several obstacles to large-scale trials remain. The real-deal plant is an endangered species. Export from Africa is illegal without proper certification, as is its import into the United States. With the approval of the South African Council for Scientific and Industrial Research, the U.K. pharmaceutical company Phytopharm was licensed in 1998 to conduct research on the plant's active ingredient. That led to commercialization partnerships with Pfizer, Inc. of New York to produce a weight-loss drug, and with the Dutch-based Unilever to develop hoodia-based foods. But both deals came apart, even after a $40 million research effort by Unilever. With no prospects for a practical, safe and effective application, Phytopharm returned all commercialization rights to South Africa.

Does that mean that products claiming to incorporate real hoodia gordonii have been banned from health food stores and internet dispensaries? Not in the very profitable and unregulated world of herbal supplements. But expect to get what you pay for, especially if you're expecting an increase in heart rate and blood pressure, headache, dizziness or nausea.

Gary Elmer, a professor of medicinal chemistry at the University of Washington, has called hoodia products one of several "fad herbals" to originate in some remote culture. "Marketers recognize they can spin this into a very profitable item." Regardless, he said, "I would think there's a pretty high element of risk with this material because we know so little."[99]

99: Sarah Jackson. "Who's Hot for Hoodia? Americans Embrace African Bushmen's Appetite Suppressant." *The Herald*, Everett, Wash., November 15, 2005.

GARCINIA CAMBOGIA

Possibly the name of a telenovela actress, but in this instance garcinia cambogia refers to a fruit native to Southeast Asia. You may have heard that it reduces appetite, improves mood, and reduces the body's ability to store fat. You may have seen it promoted by celebrity TV doctor Mehmet Oz. Perhaps you also saw Dr. Oz subsequently chewed out before a U.S. Senate consumer protection subcommittee looking at fraudulent weight-loss claims.

Real studies by real universities reviewing more than a dozen clinical trials found no important differences in weight loss between users of the supplement and other groups of men and women who were being pranked with important-looking placebo pills. Some most-advertised supplements removed the garcinia component after it was linked with potential health problems, including liver failure. That still leaves other up-and-comers in the herbal-verse, including green tea extracts, bitter orange (p-synephrine) and raspberry ketones. Again, their success at promoting weight-loss is unproven and even harder to quantify when they are combined into one shotgun "weight-loss" dietary supplement.

Products claiming to include one or more of the ingredients are widely available online and at local stores "you know and trust." Buy and try a few bottles if you envy the brief and unpleasant medical career of a lab rat.

BIG PHARMA'S BIG PLANS

Shortcuts to weight loss remain a research and business priority for Big Pharma. That's the collective, slightly demonized nickname for a dozen or so of the world's largest publicly traded pharmaceutical companies, each of which is valued at $1 billion or more.

Stockholders get sweaty under their love handles just thinking about the impact of winning FDA approval for an exclusive, new, safe, and effective diet pill, especially one that customers will have to continue taking, year after year.

"Indeed, the search for a magic bullet that can be sold to tens of millions of Americans desperate to conform to unrealistic and potentially dangerous body ideals has become a kind of Grail-like quest for the American pharmaceutical industry," as author Paul Campos described it.[100]

100: Paul, Campos. *The Obesity Myth*. New York: Gotham Books. 2004.

This would not be the first time Big Pharma has profited by convincing millions of healthy people they need to ask their doctors to prescribe an exclusive and expensive new pill to address a personal health crisis. ("Call a doctor? If I get an erection lasting more than four hours, I'm calling everyone I know!")

Critics of the Obesity Industry note that most successful weight-loss pills are able to produce, at best, a 10 percent weight loss for barely a year. That's not much for severely obese person who needs to shed 200 pounds. But it's enough to attract the typical dieter who is only mildly overweight.

"Weight-loss companies make products for people who want to look thin, not people who are concerned about their health," J. Eric Oliver said in his 2006 book, *Fat Politics*.

But any pill which attempts to override the basic metabolism and survival mechanisms of the body is likely to have dangerous, even deadly consequences. Or, as Oliver concluded, "because they convey virtually no health benefits, diet drugs are ostensibly no different from eyeliner or hair coloring — except that the latter don't have side effects like melancholy, flatulence, or heart failure."[101]

In their haste to monetize, the big drug companies have indeed rung up billions of dollars in sales — and liability claims. To their credit, regulators are taking a stricter approach to regulating anorectics, having spent years attempting to define objective measurements for both the safety and effectiveness of prescription appetite suppressants. Regulators could even be accused of dragging their heels by insisting on longer, more expansive clinical trials. Pharmaceuticals have had an equal tendency to push for speedy approval in the rush to recoup investments in research and testing. This is what has gone wrong before and can go wrong again:

PHEN-FLAM

From 1944 to 1972, certain amphetamines already approved for treatment of narcolepsy, mild depression, palsy, alcoholism, and hay fever were approved as an ancillary treatment for obesity. It was an historic first for medical treatment of a condition based solely on body weight.

101: J. Eric Oliver. *Fat Politics: The Real Story Behind America's Obesity Epidemic.* New York: Oxford University Press. 2006.

An ongoing evaluation of the minor weight-loss benefits versus the long term use of a potentially dangerous and addictive drug led the FDA, in 1977, to limit use to only a few weeks. [102]

That was enough to pull the plug. Prescriptions for the weight-loss applications of amphetamines dropped to a trickle and stayed there for 30 years.

What happened next will take its rightful place in medical malpractice history. The category includes drilling skulls to release demons and disease, or attempting to resuscitate drowning victims with a tobacco smoke enema. (True fact: This was the origin of the phrase "blowing smoke up one's __.")

In the early 1990s, as obesity was becoming more prevalent, doctors were emboldened by a single, four-year study in which 121 obese subjects were treated with either a placebo or a combination of two older drugs. They were phentermine, approved by the FDA in 1959, and fenfluramine, okayed in 1973 and marketed as Pondimin. "Although less than one third of the patients completed this study (and most regained weight during its latter stages), the findings, published in 1992, were cast in a very favorable light by the lay press, fueling the fen-phen craze," according to a 2005 review by an FDA official.[103] An estimated six million prescriptions for the fen-phen combo were written.

Although the FDA had approved the two drugs separately, their use in tandem had never been reviewed for safety or effectiveness. To this day, physicians are afforded wide latitude in prescribing drugs in combination or "off-label" — for a condition or purpose not specifically reviewed and approved by the FDA. A 2006 study reported that more than 20 percent of all drugs prescribed were for conditions not specifically approved by the FDA, and three-fourths of those (or 15 percent of *all* prescriptions) were not supported by any scientific evidence.

Off-label and on fire, the fen-phen fad spread quickly. Housewives circulated copies of the breakthrough study as if they were chain letters. Doctors who hadn't read about the study heard about it from patients. Fen-

---

102: Eric Coleman, M.D. "Anorectics on Trial: A Half Century of Federal Regulation of Prescription Appetite Suppressants." *Annals of Internal Medicine*, Vol 143, September 6, 2005. Coleman was at the time a staff physician with the FDA's Division of Metabolic and Endocrine Drug Products. His report was labeled with the disclaimer that views expressed were his own and not representing the official position of the FDA.
103: Coleman.

phen's proliferation reflected a new attitude in the medical community, one that regarded obesity as a chronic, lifelong condition which, like diabetes or high blood pressure, may require a lifelong regimen of prescription medicines.

With the patent for Pondimin (fenfluramine) about to expire in 1996, an enterprising drug company created a blend of the molecules in fen-phen. The new drug, dexfenfluramine, would be marketed as Redux. The FDA didn't get to review the original off-label recipe for fen-phen, but it would take months to consider approving this successor drug.[104]

Advisory committees were concerned by animal studies linking dexfenfluramine to nerve damage and pulmonary hypertension, an irreparable and often fatal lung disease. Advocates of the new drug argued that the animal tests were clinically irrelevant because of the high dosages used in the trials. And besides, the same drug had been widely used in Europe for years without evidence of serious damage, they argued. But the biggest rationale by Interneuron, the maker of Redux, was on the benefit side of the risk equation.

At a hearing before the FDA, the company's experts laid out a grim calculation: for every nine people who might die of taking dexfenfluramine, 280 others will be saved from an early death caused by obesity.[105] Dexfenfluramine was urgently needed, they argued, as a defense against an obesity epidemic that was going to kill hundreds of thousands of Americans a year.

Also speaking in support of Redux were representatives of a newly formed group, the American Obesity Association. Obesity is a chronic and dangerous disease, the "patient-advocate" group stressed. It did not publicize that its funding came largely from drug companies, including two involved in the Redux project.[106]

After weeks of heated debates, hand-wringing and a close vote, an FDA panel approved the sale of Redux, beginning in May 1996. It was the first new drug approved for treatment of obesity in 23 years.

Within a year, some 18 million prescriptions had been written.

104: Coleman.
105: Susan Kelleher. "Rush Toward New Weight-Loss Drugs Tramples Patients' Health." *Seattle Times*, June 26, 2005. The article was part of "Suddenly Sick," the newspaper's outstanding investigative series by Kelleher and Duff Wilson.
106: Kellerer.

Within a year and half, the risk-benefit equation had been totally wiped from the chalkboard by an unexpected and still unexplained interaction.

Reports were coming in of young women with no history of heart disease experiencing severely damaged heart valves within a few months of taking Redux. A medical clinic in Fargo, N.D. was among the first to make the connection, and forwarded two dozen cases to the Mayo Clinic in Rochester, Minnesota, which confirmed the link between heart disease and fen-phen or Redux.[107]

Evidence of the anticipated lung diseases also came to light that year, but many who took fen-phen had to wait 10 years for the damage to appear. Redux, as well as the PPA half of the fen-phen combo, were pulled from the market quickly, but not fast enough.

As the *Seattle Times* newspaper concluded in a powerful investigative piece on the power of big pharmaceutical companies and their accomplices: "In making obesity a disease, these experts helped create a billion-dollar market for the drugs that . . . killed hundreds, and damaged the hearts and lungs of tens of thousands. The story of obesity shows how it became acceptable for doctors to risk killing or injuring people on the premise that it would save them from *illnesses they might never get.*"[108]

I couldn't say it better. I only get credit for adding the italics for emphasis.

Many of the survivors of fen-phen and Redux have endured difficult surgeries for heart valve replacement or lung transplants. They are being compensated — financially, at least — by a trust fund expected to pay out more than $20 billion in legal claims.

Lessons learned? Not many. The FDA is still willing to consider new drugs that are more effective than placebos in shedding just 5 percent of body weight. And Big Pharma keeps searching for a safe and effective diet pill, along with a broader, that is, thinner, group of healthy people to take it every day.

The phentermine component of fen-phen is still legal and available by prescription, although not much in demand because of the bad company it used

---

107: Kellerer.
108: Kellerer.

to keep. Scientists say it triggers the release of certain neurotransmitters which signal a fight-or-flight response in the body, thereby blocking out hunger signals. Known side effects include increased blood pressure and heart rate, insomnia and restlessness. The recommended use is short-term, about 12 weeks. So which would you prefer -- a healthy appetite or a constant state of panic?

MERIDIA (Sibutramine)

Two months after Redux with withdrawn from the market in September 1997, the FDA approved a new drug, sibutramine, for the long-term treatment of obesity. Marketed by Abbott Laboratories in the U.S. as Meridia and in Europe as Reductil, the drug has remained waist-deep in controversy since its introduction.

The drug is believed to diminish appetite by increasing serotonin and norepinephrine levels in the brain. Sibutramine can substantially increase blood pressure and pulse in some users. Other *known* side effects include upset stomach, constipation, nausea, joint or muscle pain, sexual dysfunction and — paradoxically — increased appetite.

Opponents warned of "another diet drug disaster" but the FDA was again persuaded that its benefits — more sustained weight loss compared to placebo — outweighed the risks. But were all the risks known? In 2002, the public advocacy group Public Citizen used a Freedom of Information Act request to unearth reports of almost 400 adverse reactions to Meridia during a 43-month period. One could argue that was a small number of problems at a time when an estimated 50,000 prescriptions a month were being written. But the report obtained by Public Citizen included 19 cardiac deaths, including 10 in people under age 50. And the benefit? An additional 6 ½ pounds of weight lost per year compared to placebo, according to Public Citizen. It formally appealed to the FDA in 2002 to withdraw Meridia from the market.[109]

It took another eight years for the FDA to drop the hammer. The study that turned the tide concluded that users had a 16 percent increased risk of heart attack, stroke or death.

109: "FDA Should Immediately Ban Dangerous Diet Drug Meridia," News release, Public Citizen. March 19, 2002.

FAT BLOCKERS (AND LEAKERS)

While older prescription medicines work directly in the nervous system in an attempt to suppress appetite, the fat-blocker orlistat does its work in the colon, sometimes with embarrassing proof that it's working. With side effects that include diarrhea, flatulence or a greasy discharge, it's not surprising that prescriptions for the drug, marketed by Roche Pharma as Xenical, took a nosedive soon after the first round of desperate dieters got to the bottom of the problem.

Brown sounds notwithstanding, the brass at London-based GlaxoSmithKline heard the jingle of cash registers, agreeing to pay Sweden's Roche Holding $100 million and a share of future profits for the U.S. rights to introduce a half-strength, over-the-counter version called alli (and modestly spelled with a lowercase "a").

The FDA approved prescription Xenical in 1999 and agreed to the commercialized over-the-counter version in early 2007. The basic arguments over risk and benefits were the same in both cases, although the FDA had to be convinced that no serious harm would come to those who would be foolish enough to take more than the recommended dosage of three pills a day, one before each meal.

I won't make a habit of quoting anonymous Internet sources, but this comment posted under a financial page story about the introduction of alli would make a compelling warning label: "This is VERY important," wrote Amy, a nurse practitioner who used Xenical for seven years -- and prescribed it to several patients. "You will LEAK orange foul-smelling oil from your tushy if you eat fatty food! It will not clean with toilet paper, it will stain the toilet bowl until scrubbed with bleach, and it will leak THROUGH your pants uncontrollably, also staining your clothes. This will happen only once to convince you to decrease your fat intake . . . lol. No fast food on this medicine, no greasy foods, no pizza especially." She advises anyone starting the drug to carry baby wipes and an extra pair of pants until they learn the rules.[110]

Users are also advised to take vitamin supplements to offset the fat-soluble nutrients blocked by the orlistat.

110: Amy's comment was posted under a May 9, 2007 article by Eric Buscemi at bloggingstocks.com titled "New Obesity Drug the Real Deal?"

NEW DRUGS, OLD WARNINGS

The prize money for an anti-obesity drug worth billions in potential life-long prescriptions is forever tempting. So Big Pharma keeps spending millions on the entry fees in the form of laboratory research, clinical trials and lobbying U.S. and foreign regulators for approval. Following below are the newest drugs to enter the ring.[111] Which ones will still be standing in a few years? Perhaps the real question is how many severe or unexpected side effects must be discovered to deal a knockout punch.

Marketed as Contrave, this one combines naltrexone, which is used to treat alcohol and opioid dependence, with bupropion, an antidepressant said to reduce weight gain in those who are trying to quit smoking. Add up the combined possible side effects and ask yourself if you also crave nausea, constipation, headache, vomiting, dizziness, increased heart rate, blood pressure and risk of seizures or suicidal thoughts and behaviors. This, to me, sounds eerily similar to a night of heavy drinking capped by a round of Russian roulette.

Lorcaserin, brand-name Belviq, is intended to decrease appetite and increase feelings of fullness. Possible side effects include headache, nausea, dry mouth, dizziness, fatigue and constipation. Perhaps I should say these are the side effects you would prefer. The drug's formula raised some concerns because it works somewhat like fenfluramine. But, as of late 2015, there is no evidence Belviq will damage the heart, according to health educators at Mayo Clinic. Still, the drug may increase heart rate -- something users will need to monitor closely.

We'll know Big Pharma has run out of crazy names to copyright when they have to steal the name of Superman's impish villain, Mr. Mxyzptlk. Here's another new one called Qsymia, although it's just a combination of two older drugs. It falls back on the stimulant phentermine to curb appetite, coupled with the anti-migraine and -seizure drug topiramate. Separately, the drugs offer any combination of insomnia, dry mouth, dizziness and constipation. Together, they increase the risk of birth defects. So Qsymia is off limits to any woman crazy enough to attempt weight loss during pregnancy.

Saxenda (from the Latin, meaning "Quit playing that damn saxophone"),

---

111: "Prescription Weight-Loss Drugs." mayoclinic.org. April 30, 2015.

is a double dose of a liraglutide, a treatment for Type 2 diabetes. Side effects include nausea, vomiting and pancreatitis. But you don't care because, unlike all the others which are taken orally, Saxenda requires a once-daily injection. And it costs about $1,000 per month.

Taking any of these drugs requires more than a willingness to accept the potential consequences. Until Big Pharma can find a way around it, their valuable customers are going to need a doctor's prescription. A good physician is not the one who writes up whatever you request. A good doctor will consider your weight, BMI, health, other medications, and whether weight loss has any real benefit beyond losing five pounds for an upcoming event. A great doctor cares enough to just say no.

And what if there really was a pill to make weight loss easier? How many months or years of interfering with normal human metabolism could be reliably safe? And how many of us would bother with a healthy diet and fitness habits if the atonement for slacking off came 90 to a bottle?

09

METABOLISM

DIETS FAIL, NATURE PREVAILS

After being frightened with perhaps too much information about popular weight-loss prescriptions and various impotent potions, you may have jettisoned your own stash into the toilet. Good riddance. Except for the powerful drain on your pocketbook and patience, all weight-loss interventions are feeble machinations against one of the most powerful forces on earth — your body's own sophisticated defenses against biological change in general and starvation in particular. Remember, as was described in Chapter 4, your body is genetically programmed to protect your natural weight range against all manner of attackers. Perhaps you are feeling empowered by a new prescription appetite suppressant or motivated to slim down for a wedding in three months and have a personal trainer standing by to slap cookies out of your hand. "Zatso? Bring it on!" your body says. And 19 times out of 20, the body will win. Newer scientific studies are adding more detail to our understanding of the processes at the molecular level, but the big picture remains unchanged: from our parents all the way back to our Cro-magnon roots, our genetic histories, determine how bodies process sugars and fats, feelings of hunger and satiety and, most importantly here, our natural body weight. "You were not built to lose weight," as one obesity researcher describes it. "You were built to not starve to death."[112]

112: Seeley, Randy J. , Ph.D., currently Associate Director of the Obesity Research Center at the University of Cincinnati, as quoted in "Leptin's Legacy" by David Tenenbaum, HHMI (*Howard Hughes Medical Institute*) Bulletin, March 2003.

HOME, HOME IN THE RANGE

Few of us have or will face starvation, but the same forces that support *homeostasis* -- the body's preference for a relatively stable equilibrium -- also enforce boundaries against sudden weight gain or loss. Each of us is believed to have a natural *set point* in the middle of a natural range of 10 to 20 pounds. Your job is to *find your* weight and defend it.

Researchers don't really have a way to pinpoint an individual's weight at set point. However, some believe most of us are at that point after at least a year of mindful, drama-free eating and consistent, moderate activity. By then, sudden weight gain or loss outside the body's natural range will be met with stiff metabolic and hormonal resistance.

You might quickly lose 10 pounds by trimming calories, but be ready to hit a plateau where the same or greater effort can't take the weight any lower. Your metabolism will slow, your body temperature will drop, you'll sleep more and wake up insatiably hungry.

A fair analogy is your body temperature. Not everyone has a "normal" temperature of 98.6 degrees Fahrenheit, but when infection or environmental conditions push body temperature up or down, several inherit defense mechanisms will join forces to reclaim normality, or die trying. Are you listening, or trying not to hear? Extreme, prolonged or repeated efforts to lose more weight than your body can tolerate is physically unhealthy and emotionally damning. Extreme weight-loss dieting and overdone exercise is immediately dangerous and ultimately fruitless.

So sad. So discouraging, you're thinking.

Oh, boohoo, your body replies. It was trying hard to make you listen all along.

You just chose not to hear. Or blamed yourself for each try and fail.

So now what?

A personal, fatsmart rebirth. That's what!

Most of us still have ample power to *maintain* our current weight or, with just a little more effort, reach the lower range limit of set point — slowly, healthily, happily, and for many years to come. We don't need a weight-loss diet. We need a healthy diet that allows for modest, persistent weight loss.

At this point, a typical diet book would introduce some contrived theories and labels such as "the EuroHollywood MetaboRific DynaCarb Response" in an effort to convince you that I, your generous author, am about to share for the trifling cost of one mass-marketed volume a collection of great weight-loss secrets never before disclosed at any price. In typical fashion, I would go on to pad this book about "breakthrough discoveries" which are actually a new spin on a lot of old, forgotten, or disproven science. I would say as little as possible about the need for regular exercise. I would stress my credentials, but cover my butt by telling you to consult your physician before acting on anything I've written. (Well, actually I *am* telling you that.)

And lastly I would imply that any failures you experience in applying my findings are solely the result of your own sloth and weak will.[113] It's your fault. That's the diet book routine, is it not? That said, I am hesitant even to suggest that you trust me. And so, on the delicate subject on dieting and weight control, I am asking that you place your trust *not* in me but where it safely belongs.

- Trust your DNA: Whether by intelligent design or cosmic happenstance, the survival of humanity is partly dependent on the body's stubborn retention of fat borne nutrients.

- Trust your appetite: Pay attention when your stomach says you're hungry and when you're full.

- Trust your taste buds: 10,000 of them can't be wrong.

- Trust yourself. Family, friends, clocks, and advertising are always telling you when and what to eat. Tell them that if you're hungry, you'll eat whatever you want.

REVENGE OF THE CHEESE STEAK

Any snakes, lizards or other cold-blooded ectotherms reading along may skip this part because it doesn't apply to them. The rest of us endotherms, i.e.

113: William Bennett, M.D. and Joel Gurin. *The Dieter's Dilemma: Eating Less and Weighing More.* New York: Basic Books, Inc., 1982. The book's tongue-in-cheek advice on "How to Write Your Own Diet Book," pp.227-231, was on target in 1982 and the formula has been copied hundreds of times since.

all mammals and birds, will continue to sweat or shiver as needed to maintain a constant body temperature. Temperature regulation is just one of several homeostatic mechanisms carried out in the background. While our brains concentrate on more important things, like an hour of hardcore food porn courtesy of "Diners, Drive-Ins and Dives," our bodies are still in the real world. Homeostatic feedback loops continuously monitor and adjust hormone levels, blood glucose and acidity levels -- anything affecting body fat and weight levels.

Let's say you recently managed to achieve a personal-best weight loss of 18 pounds in just a few weeks on a popular crash diet. Congratulations: you've probably lost about 13 pounds of water and some very important muscle tissue. You may be proud, but your body, sensing a nasty famine in the outside world, is going into panic mode. Your resting metabolic rate is dropping by as much as 45 percent in order to conserve energy.

Weight loss is halted, but pounced to rebound as soon as you grab the keys to the SUV and head down to your local diner for your own, richly deserved Philly cheese steak with onion rings. You just need a break to let your willpower heal, you think. And in a couple of weeks, you're back to where you started (if you're lucky) or maybe a few pounds heavier. The maddening, unnecessary weight cycle is complete. You've sacrificed foods you love to achieve an unrealistic goal, then felt deprived, succumbed and gorged, and piled on the guilt.

Just be glad you're an amateur at this weight-loss foolishness.

THE BIGGEST LOSERS (AND GAINERS)

At least you didn't have to torture and humiliate yourself in front of 8 million of your countrymen. For 17 seasons, NBC's "The Biggest Loser" presented a pseudo-reality competition among dozens of morbidly obese men and women. They endured both a starvation diet and exaggerated boot camp exercises in pursuit of a cash prize and a misplaced desire to prove their inner worth to friends and family. Viewers who brought some combination of empathy and sadism to the spectacle were treated to the site of trainers screaming at participants soaked in their own sweat and tears, then briefly buoyed by contestants weighing in while nearly naked. Some got to pose proudly with their comically fat "before" jeans. Most succeeded at substantial weight loss-- for a while.

After each season finale, the rest of us were left to wonder how many of the big losers would be able to maintain their big losses, and for how long. But only one of us saw an opportunity to conduct a thorough scientific study that would be considered too cruel to conduct under any other circumstances. He was Kevin Hall, Ph.D., a diet and metabolism specialist within the National Institutes of Health. Hall and his team made arrangements with the 16 "Biggest Loser" candidates from Season 8 to undergo a thorough analysis of their weight and body fat composition, resting metabolic rate, and blood chemistry. That work began just before the competition began and provided the baseline for a follow-up analysis at the conclusion of the 30-week competition in December 2009. Revealing, to be sure! More importantly to understanding the body's response to intentional weight loss, the researchers persuaded all but two of the 16 -- six men and eight women -- to undergo the clinical examination again six years later.[114]

The documented changes in blood chemistry were the biggest revelation, but I'm guessing most readers would skip directly to the tale of the scales. So here goes:

The average pre-competition contestant weight was a hefty 328 pounds. Thirty tired, hungry and dehydrated weeks later, they had lost an average of 128.5 pounds to reach 199.7 pounds. Bravo! They lost dang near 200 pounds, or 39 percent of their "before" weights. That's like a 250-pound person dropping to 152 pounds, or a 152-pounder shriveling to a boney 92.

And so, during the five years and 22 weeks after the TV lights dimmed on bodies draped in folds of excess skin, they tried to keep the weight off. They tried hard, many of them exercising several hours a day while strictly limiting calories. And they were always hungry. They often succumbed to the eating binges and bouts of guilt and self-loathing experienced every Ding Dong day by millions of weight-loss amateurs. Keeping the weight off, they learned, wasn't merely as hard as losing it. It was harder, in terms of will power, because there was no endgame, no finish line, no pot of gold, and no redemption. And it was physically impossible, because their own bodies organized agonizing, powerful, and unending acts of sabotage.

114: Erin Fothergill, Kevin D. Hall and others. "Persistent Metabolic Adaptation 6 Years After 'The Big-gest Loser'." *Obesity* (journal) August 2016.

After six years, each contestant had regained, on average, 90.4 pounds. About 70 percent of their hard-won weight loss had disappeared. Compared to their starting weight of 328 pounds, the Biggest Losers averaged 290 pounds after six years. Average net weight loss: 38 pounds -- a paltry 11.5 percent less than their weight when they embarked on the world's most conspicuous intentional weight loss program.[115]

THE UNFORGOTTEN FAMINE

Blood tests, however, revealed a more significant change over which they had no control. Their resting metabolic rate -- a measure of normal caloric burn without any activity -- dropped as expected during the 30-week contest, from an average of about 2,600 calories down to barely 2,000 a day. That's what our bodies do when faced with a famine, whether the setting is a third-world dust bowl or a Los Angeles television studio.

What shocked the researchers was that contestants' *metabolic rates did not rebound*, even as the pounds came back. Six years after they had regained 70 percent of their original weight loss, average resting metabolic rates had dropped further, down to 1,900 calories a day. It was as if their bodies could not forget the terrible famine from six years ago and were now better prepared to face a new and harsher round of starvation.

The drop in RMR would be borderline fair to the contestants if their hunger subsided proportionately. It did, but not for long. To objectively measure hunger, researchers relied on blood test taken before, after, and long after the competition. They looked at leptin, the so-called satiety hormone produced by fat cells to help regulate energy balance by telling your brain: "We're good. Stop eating." Contestants started the dieting ordeal with an average leptin concentration of 41.16 nanograms per milliliter. That means ... Well, it doesn't matter. Just know that it was appropriate for their weight levels. But 30 weeks of rapid fat loss made a strong impression on the fat cells. Leptin levels plummeted to nearly nothing -- just 2.56 ng/m. Without leptin, the hunger hormone ghrelin had no opposing force. The contestants were very damn hungry at all times. No surprise there, although researchers were happy to have the hard data to explain it.

115: Fothergill.

In the remaining five-plus years of the study, the biggest losers exercised and followed low-calorie diets, but they remained hungry. Binges and backsliding were inevitable and the weight came back. So did their leptin levels, but only to 27.68 ng/mL, or about two-thirds of their baseline concentrations of the satiety hormone. Just to maintain their weight loss, the contestants had to forgo hundreds of calories a day compared to a non-dieter the same size.

Contestants were somewhat relieved to learn their metabolic adaptation and satiety hormones had conspired against them. Some felt cheated, like the 36-year-old pastor from Charlotte, N.C., who had returned to his original 444 pounds and was still gaining. "It's kind of like learning you have a life sentence," he said.[116]

Investigators could offer little encouragement to millions of others trying to maintain a significant weight loss. "As long as you are below your original weight," said Dr. Michael Schwartz, an obesity researcher not involved in the study, "your body is going to try to get you back."[117]

FINN TWINS AND LESSER LOSERS

The study of "The Biggest Losers" was both dramatic and weighty because of its revelations about metabolic adjustment and hunger hormones. It was among the recent projects to push peer-reviewed science beyond the anecdotal evidence that intensive dieting is not only fraught with futility, but capable of *permanently sabotaging future efforts to control weight.*

Perhaps now you are wondering (and hoping) if the extremes of "The Biggest Loser" experiment are irrelevant to weight-loss amateurs. Is set point science more forgiving of frequent attempts to maintain a more modest intentional weight loss?

Let me briefly sidestep the answer by punting to a group of Finnish researchers. The Finns have maintaining a large database of twins -- male and female, identical and fraternal -- that is extremely useful in any effort to suss out genetic influences. The study we care about was published in 2012 and gathered

---

116: Kolata, Gina. "After 'The Biggest Loser,' Their Bodies Fought To Regain Weight." New York Times. May 2, 2016. Kolata is a senior medical writer for The New York Times and detailed the results of other weight studies in one of her nine books, *Rethinking Thin: The New Science of Weight Loss-- and the Myths and Realities of Dieting.*

117: Kolata.

information from more than 4,000 individual twins at ages 16, 17, 18 and 25.

Researchers collected data on weight, eating and dieting habits, and also controlled for variables such as gender, physical activity, smoking, economic status, parents' BMI and frequency of breakfast eating.[118] Yes, they believe a good breakfast is *that* important.

At age 25, each was asked how many times had they had intentionally lost 5 kilograms (11 pounds) or more of weight.

The verdict: Study participants with no history of weight-loss dieting had the least amount of weight gain. The "reward" for those who tried dieting five or more times was the largest average weight gain between ages 16 and 25. And twins with a history of intentional weight loss were heavier at all ages than their brothers and sisters who never attempted weight loss.

The weight differences weren't huge. Heck, the participants were just 25 years old. But the findings were consistent enough for the Finns to conclude that frequent intentional weight loss renders "dieters prone to future weight gain . . . independent of genetic factors." [119]

In summary: bicycling, good; unicycling, best left to circus performers; weight cycling, bad.

To this, I want to add a reminder that dieting can be especially dangerous for children. Teenagers and preteens who diet to extremes risk not getting the nutrients required for normal body growth. Children who bring unhealthy, adult-like anxieties to dieting possibly have psychological problems which warrant medical intervention.

We just can't pooh-pooh this much black and white science about metabolism, dieting and health. Still, there is room for more comforting and colorful reasons to abandon weight-loss diets. Here are several good ones, as presented with feminist perspective by a pioneering grassroots advocacy organization, the Council on Size & Weight Discrimination:[120]

118: K.H. Pietiläinen and others. "Does Dieting Make You Fat? A Twin Study." *International Journal of Obesity.* © 2012 Macm'tillan Publishers Ltd.
119: Pietiläinen.
120: "Top Ten Reasons to Give Up Dieting," © 1994 Council on Size & Weight Discrimination. cswd.org.

- Diets don't work and can end with more weight gained that lost. Diets are expensive, especially those that require special diet products. Diets are boring and encourage food fixations that cast a shadow over everything else in life.

- Diets don't necessarily improve your health and can actually cause health problems and lead to eating disorders. Dieting can make you afraid of food, robbing you of energy, pleasure, comfort and nourishment.

- Diets don't make you beautiful. Diets are not sexy. "Very few people will ever look like models. Glamour is a look, not a size. You don't have to be thin to be attractive," the activists say.

- "Learning to love and accept yourself just as you are will give you self-confidence, better health, and a sense of well-being that will last a lifetime," the group believes.

HOPE FOR THE HOPELESS

To be perfectly clear, most of the health concerns described above apply to frequent or extreme weight-loss dieting. You'll need to consult with several medical and nutrition specialists to define "frequent" or "extreme" as it applies to you, your weight and other personal health risks.

Gradual, healthy weight loss is often recommended and achievable. Be forewarned that basic metabolic and hormonal changes resulting from a weight loss of 10 percent of more can persist as long as six years, according to Dr. Holly Lofton, a weight management specialist at New York University's Langone Medical Center. With the help of medication, she says about half of her patients are able to manage their imbalance of hunger and satiety hormones in order to achieve and maintain a weight loss.[121]

Moving to a new, lower set point and weight range is the backbone of the process. Topping Lofton's recommendations in that regard is having protein at every meal and snack. Muscle tissue burns more calories than fat. The protein fights hunger and minimizes loss of muscle during weight loss, she says.

121: Susan Rinkunas. "Why, Exactly, Do Our Bodies Fight Us On Weight Loss" thecut.com. May 13, 2016.

She recommends cardiovascular exercise for patients until they're halfway to a weight-loss goal. The cardio burns fat and minimizes the frustrating weight gain that comes with strength training. After the midpoint, she increases resistance exercises to regain lost muscle and prepare for maintenance.[122]

Lofton and her colleagues recommend a diet of whole foods. No surprise there considering that processed foods are higher in sugars and artificial sweeteners that are easily digested without controlling hunger.

In Chapter 12, we'll look at a painless alternative to weight-loss dieting. It's rated M for Mature. It's nothing nasty – just a method that requires the maturity to distinguish between a craving for potassium-rich foods and jonesing for a pint of butter pecan ice cream.

122: Rinkunas.

10

FATS AND CARBS

L et's just believe Joan Rivers was trying to share her knowledge of good nutrition when she let it slip that Elizabeth Taylor had pierced her ears. And gravy came out.

Dietary fats — the kind we put in our mouths — are not the same thing as body fat, but the relationship between the two is one of endless hand-wringing, research and debate. There's been a lot of fiber in the news about unhealthy fats and carbohydrates and their impact on coronary disease. Let's see if we have a dog in this fight.

Fats in food are digested and chemically transformed before becoming blood-borne fat cells. Fat cells come in several categories. Let's think in exaggerated terms. What would you prefer in your arteries: light, fluid oils, or fats that are thick at room temperature, such as lard, shortening, butter, and most margarines?

Poly- and monounsaturated fats are both *un*saturated fats. They're found in most vegetable oils, including oils from olive, canola, corn and soybean. They're also found in some fish and nuts including salmon, trout, herring and walnuts. Sound healthy? Pretty much!

Saturated fat is found mostly in animal products. Beef, pork, lamb, lard, butter, cream, whole milk and cheese are all good sources of flavor and, yes, saturated fat. There are also a few plants famous for their saturated fats, those being the so-called tropical oils -- coconut, palm and palm kernel.

And finally, there are *trans* fats. These occur naturally in foods such as . . . Umm. None at all. Instead, they are food-like substances created by corporate food scientists principally motivated to lower production costs and increase shelf life, since each contributes to profitability.

TRANSFORMATIVE TRANS FATS

Basically, trans fats are liquid oils that have been transformed into solids through a century-old molecule shuffling process pioneered in Germany. It's called hydrogenation. Procter & Gamble acquired the U.S. rights in 1909 and quickly introduced the first partially hydrogenated shortening. Paired with free recipe booklets, Crisco became a huge success. About the same time, shortages of butter and a surplus of soybean oil opened the pantry door for partially hydrogenated margarine.

Legislators from dairy states fought back for decades by pushing for margarine to be sold in its natural, lardy-looking white state or, worse, colored pink. Some state laws with such restrictions still remain on the books as unenforced novelties. Margarine steadily replaced butter in the Western diet beginning in the 1950s, when television advertising churned out messages touting the butter substitute's health, cost and flavor benefits, whether real or imaginary.

Over the course of a century, trans fats transformed home cooking, restaurant kitchens, commercial bakeries, and food manufacturing. But pesky nutritionists kept asking if it was appropriate to fool Mother Nature. They knew right away that trans fats, unlike other dietary fats, are not essential to good health. Some recent studies suggest a link between trans fat consumption and an increase in cancers of the prostate and breast. Infertility and liver dysfunction also may be aggravated by heavy intake of trans fats. On the other hand, studies linking trans fats to diabetes have been contradictory or inconclusive.

Researchers are pretty gee-darn certain, however, about trans fat's contribution to coronary heart disease. Like saturated fat, trans fat has a nasty habit of increasing blood levels of low-density lipoprotein, better known as LDL, the so-called "bad" cholesterol. At the same time, trans fats lower the HDL, or "good" cholesterol in the blood. So that's double bad, like deep-fried Twinkies. Oh, and trans fat may increase the inflammation that promotes fatty blockages in blood vessels. (If you get your good and bad HDLs and LDLs confused, like I do, remember: H for happy; L for lousy. Or H and L for high and low, which is where you want those numbers to be.)

As early as 1994, the American Journal of Public Health was warning that trans fat may be to blame in 30,000 deaths per year and, of course, many more cases of nonfatal coronary disease.[123] And researchers in Boston and the Netherlands concluded in 2006 that on a per-calorie basis and even at low levels of consumption (1 to 3 percent of total energy intake) trans fats confer a substantially increased risk of heart disease. That 1 to 3 percent could be a measly 20 to 60 calories per day for someone taking in 2,000 calories per day.[124]

The following year, a Harvard School of Public Health study independently concluded that women in the U.S. with the highest levels of trans fats in their blood have three times the risk of heart disease as their sisters with the least amount.[125] That is certainly a consideration for anyone, male or female, predisposed to or already dealing with cardiovascular disease.

Yeah, yeah. Who wants to live forever just to see Pet Rocks, leisure suits and "10-4, Good Buddy" come back in style? *Fat, Smart and Happy* Nation wants to know: Do trans fats put the fat on me? A group of 42, civic-minded male African green monkeys volunteered to find out.

Getting together for meals at Wake Forest University School of Medicine for six years (equivalent to about 20 human years), the group enjoyed a diet carefully controlled to meet their busy monkey energy requirements without promoting weight gain. They all enjoyed the same number of calories each day, with 35 percent of calories coming from fat. But half of the test monkeys got 8 percent of their calories from trans fat -- comparable to people who eat a lot of fast foods -- while the others received those calories as monounsaturated fat, such as olive oil. Did it matter?

Yes. Big time. The monkeys on a fatty American-style diet put on the pounds, averaging a 7.2 percent increase in body weight, compared to a 1.8

123: Walter C. Willett, MD, DrPH, and Albert Ascherio, MD, DrPH."Trans Fatty Acids: Are the Effects Only Marginal?" *The American Journal of Public Health*. 1994.
124: Dariush Mozaffarian, MD and others. "Trans Fatty Acids and Cardiovascular Disease." *The New England Journal of Medicine*. 2006.
125: Qi Sun, MD, and others. "A Prospective Study of Trans Fatty Acids in Erythrocytes and Risk of Coronary Heart Disease." *Circulation (Journal of the American Heart Association)*. 2007.

percent swelling among the more Mediterranean-style monkeys. The monkeys fed trans fats were further embarrassed by CT scans which confirmed that most of their extra fat was deposited in their abdomens, giving them the apple shape strongly associated with diabetes and heart disease in humans.[126]

You don't have to be a lab animal to monkey around with dangerous amounts of trans fat. Baked goods such as pie, cake, cookies, Danish or doughnuts have long averaged 2 to 4 grams per serving. Crackers, pancakes, French fries, enchiladas and breaded chicken nuggets are also a reliable source of trans fats. Don't be lulled into unhealthy complacency by packaging that declares "No Trans Fats." Although a large majority of popular fast foods and snacks have been weaned of trans fats in the past decade, most are still loaded with added fats, including sludgy saturated fats.

In January 2006, the U.S. Food and Drug Administration required the food industry to declare the amount of trans fat in food on the Nutrition Facts label. Since then, many processed foods and restaurant staples have been reformulated to reduce the amount of partially hydrogenated oils (PHO) responsible for most trans fat. As more nutritionists and policy-makers came on board, the FDA took a bigger step in November 2015, removing its "generally recognized as safe" status for PHOs.

An outright ban on the artificial trans fat took effect June 18, 2018. Still, the FDA is allowing foods produced before that date to "work their way through distribution" (and your arteries) through all of 2019. Good riddance.

LABELS AND OTHER LIES

When it comes to foods, oil equals fat and fat equals calories. Too bad we can't rely on those government-mandated nutrition labels to say so. Look at the bewildering selection of cooking oils on grocery shelves and you'll find oils made from olives, peanuts, canola (rapeseed) or soybeans, although the latter is always labeled "vegetable oil." All of them, even the "light" olive oils, contain the same number of calories -- 9 per gram, or 120 per tablespoon. And yet, there it is: A can of spray oil boldly labeled "FAT-FREE!"

126: "Trans Fat Leads To Weight Gain Even On Same Total Calories, Animal Study Shows." Wake Forest University Baptist Medical Center news release, June 19, 2006. *www.sciencedaily.com.*

Perhaps the spray contains graphite, a popular lubricant every bit as tasty as pencil lead. Nope, it's oil. Because of unsavory interactions between food lobbyists, Congress and the Food and Drug Administration, anything less than a half-gram of fat per serving doesn't have to be listed on nutrition labels. You can do that math, but it won't make sense. In FDA-speak, .49 grams of fat equals zero grams of fat.

When reading package nutrition labels, look first for the "servings per container" and don't be surprised if what looks likes a reasonable amount for one serving is listed as two or more portions. This common practice makes the labeled amounts for calories, fats and carbohydrates look more acceptable than they really are. Even more deceptive is a common snack industry practice of generously wrapping up a serving that is actually 5 to 50 percent heavier than the net weight listed on the package. It's hard to complain about that, I reckon. But nutrition labels only reflect the minimum net weight. Use an ounce and a half of caution if you're tracking fat grams.

Packaging that honestly touts a low *percentage* of fat can be misleading, too, because serving sizes and total grams of fat are really what matters. Whole milk has "only" 3.5 percent fat, but that's 8 grams in an 8-ounce glass, 16 grams in a pint. You might rather have a 3-ounce scoop of ice cream, with just 5 grams of fat.

Some packaging claims actually mean something. Low-fat means 3 grams of fat or less per serving; reduced fat means a fourth less fat than regular products (whatever "regular" means); light or "lite" means 50 percent or less fat or calories.

Most importantly, don't equate fat-free with calorie-free. Soft drinks, fruit juice, beer, booze, sugar, hard candy, even the delicious chocolate syrup I've been known to chug straight from the bottle -- all are fat-free and still loaded with calories.

GOOD AND BETTER FATS

All this *CSI: Dietary Fat* stigmatizes an important food group that still deserves a place at the table. You wouldn't want a flashlight without a reliable battery any more than a body without an efficient energy storage system. Body fat protects important organs, helps dilute dangerous toxins in the blood stream and to regulate body temperature. Healthy hair and skin requires dietary fat, as does the normal functioning of body cells. Important vitamins A, D, E and K can only be absorbed and used with the help of fat.

So eat fats! Be at least a little fat yourself! Just pay as much attention to quantity and quality as you would when choosing a skin moisturizer or motor oil. And don't believe everything you've been hearing, even if it sounds healthy. In its highly recommended (by me, at least) monthly newsletter, *Consumer Reports On Health* rounded up the latest research on dietary fats and popped some Conventional Wisdom balloons in the process.

The CW says olive and canola oils are the healthiest, primarily because they contain mostly monounsaturated fats, valued for lowering lousy (LDL) cholesterol without lowering happy (HDL) cholesterol. But *Consumer Reports* says polyunsaturated oils such as those derived from corn, sunflower and fish may have an overall better influence on heart health, even though the research which suggests it doesn't explain why.

Furthermore, very low-fat diets may not be heart healthiest, because they also reduce good HDL levels. What about cancer? *Consumer Reports'* review of the data suggests that limiting fat intake may benefit people who already have breast or prostate cancer, but for most others, fat intake doesn't seem to promote or prevent cancers.

Wait. I hear you, Fat Nation. Isn't cutting back on fats still the best way to maintain or lose weight? Well, no more so than cutting carbs and sugars. It's The Calories, Stupid. Yes, fats are loaded with 'em, about 9 per gram versus 4 calories per gram of protein or carbohydrates.

"But fatty foods usually contain protein," *Consumer Reports* reminds us, "and that combination makes you feel fuller longer (whereas) very low-fat diets can be hard to maintain." [127]

Remember that healthy foods can lose their advantages in a hurry. A whole potato weighing 3 ounces has no fat and only 65 calories. Convert that to 3 ounces of small-cut French fries and you've got 15 grams of fat and 265 calories.

127: "The New Facts About Fats: What You Think You Know Might Need To Be Revised," *Consumer Reports on Health*. October 2007.

Sounds incredible until we get to 3 ounces of potato chips, somehow enriched to 30 grams of fat and 450 salt-encrusted calories. And from chips to hips? You better believe it.

Avoid fast-food favorites. A Big Mac will cost you 28 grams of fat, including 10 grams of saturated fat. Or you could think of that as health food if you chose it over Hardee's 2/3-pound Monster Thickburger with 90 fat grams (33 grams saturated).

Be just as careful with those slow-food favorites. Menu words such as buttered, French fried, breaded, scalloped, au gratin, or creamy are just a more-appetizing way of saying "dripping with fat." Put your waiter on the spot by asking about the types of oils used in the kitchen.

Remove the skin from poultry before eating or, better, before cooking. This cuts fat by more than half. Ditto for trimming visible fats from steaks and chops.

Don't come home from the grocery with bags of salty, fried, or cheesy snacks. Instead, bring home a colorful mix of fresh fruits and vegetables. Prep them right away, so they'll be the first thing on the refrigerator shelf when you go rummaging for a snack.

Steam, broil, or roast meat, fish, and poultry. Use a little spray oil or vegetable oil for skillet dinners. Do not mimic the TV chefs who pour on a half-cup of oil and call it a "drizzle." Olive oil is perfect for a saute, salad dressing, or marinade. Canola oil is well suited to baking.

I don't feel bad about keeping genuine whole milk on hand for coffee, recipes or the occasional full glass required with cookies or a peanut butter sandwich. Whole milk has 4.6 grams of saturated fat per serving, versus only 1.5 grams with 1 percent milk. And there is twice as much cholesterol in the whole milk. But the protein and carbohydrates are the same, regardless of content. If you've had a hard time switching from whole milk to low-fat milk, suffer through a few days of drinking 1 percent or skimmed no-fat milk. After that, the 2 percent milk will taste super creamy.

CARBOHYDRATES

Fatty foods are like real love. They have the ability to break your heart, but also to nurture the body and soul. Fat satisfies the palate and subdues hunger.

An affair with carbohydrates, however, is more like a one-night stand. In their simplest, least nutritious form, carbohydrates are merely snacks that make you keep coming back for more. "They are culinary pornography," says William Leith, the British wordsmith whose binge battles were described in Chapter 6. In his experience, potato chips equal *Penthouse*. "Eating carbohydrate snacks is not exactly having a meaningful relationship with food," Leith writes. "Fill yourself with snacks, and you'll feel empty a couple of hours later." [128]

Sugars, starches, and fiber all find a home in the blended family nutritionists classify as carbohydrates. Like the fat family, the carbohydrate clan is large enough to encompass a range of over-achievers and ne'er-do-wells. The goldbrick carbs are the type most encountered in fast foods, vending machines, and the inner aisles of grocery stores. Lazy carbs are the simple or highly refined carbohydrates such as table sugar, corn syrup, white flour and the thousands of varieties of breads, pasta, cakes, candy, chips, and soft drinks made with them.

Complex carbs are like the smart uncle or older sister who knows a lot, but doesn't give it away all at once. They're more likely to be found at the farmers' market or along the produce aisle. They are considered complex because of their long, intertwined molecular structures, but are still simply delicious in the form of countless fruits, vegetables and whole grains. Actually, the carbs in fruits are also simple, but because they come with so many valuable nutrients, they're welcome at any gathering of healthy foods.

Overall, carbohydrates are just recovering from the hysteria of 2003-2004 when millions of dieters embraced the low-carbohydrate "revolution" popularized by the late Dr. Robert Atkins. Atkins believed -- and recent studies have corroborated -- that sugar, flour, high-fructose corn syrup, and other refined carbohydrates were to blame for increasing rates of obesity. Many dieters embraced the concept without reading the fine print. They just jumped at the opportunity for a daily breakfast of steak and eggs, with heavy servings of fats

---

128: William Leith. *Confessions of a Food Addict.* New York: *Gotham Books*, 2005.

and meats throughout the day but only token amounts of the salad greens and vegetables Atkins also recommended.

During the first and strictest of the four stages in the Atkins diet, rigid adherents were sometimes saddled with headaches, muscle weakness, irritable bowels and a metallic taste in the mouth signaling the onset of their body's fat-burning ketosis. That's because consuming less than 150 grams of carbohydrates per day can also deprive the body of sufficient glucose for normal tissue repair. Regardless, the Atkins acolytes were numerous enough for a time to push down sales of rice and pasta and to force bakeries to devise new brands of tasteless low-carb breads.

Yes, the Atkins army lost weight for a few months, some longer, but eventually the craze was neutered by conflicting medical studies about its impact on heart disease, and because the diet was expensive to maintain. And, even with its tolerance for meats, poultry and seafood, it was *borrriiinng*. Food porn doesn't get any more seductive than a buttery baked potato or fresh yeast roll to the person who hasn't had one for a month. Regardless of which foods are allowed and which are censored, we know nearly all dieters will be back at their starting weight within two years.

Looking back, many nutritionists believe the any weight loss experienced by low-carb dieters had more to do with their uptake in protein, which is bulky and satisfying enough to keep hunger at bay for several hours. But the same low-carbers who skimped on grains, fruits and vegetables may not have gotten sufficient fiber and vitamins. [129]

THE GI BILL OF HEALTH

Anyone already dealing with the difficulties of diabetes, or just trying to avoid dangerously high blood-glucose levels, already knows that grains and vegetables are valued for their low GI, or glycemic index. GI is a trusted scale that reflects how quickly carbohydrates break down in digestion and release glucose into the blood over a two-hour period. The index uses glucose itself as the high reference point, assigning it a value of 100. High GI foods are plentiful

129: Daniel J. DeNoon. "Low-Carb Diets Work, But Safety Still An Issue." *WebMD Health News*. Sept. 2, 2004. Interview with Arne Astrup, MD, PhD, nutritionist and head of the Institute of Human Nutrition at the Centre of Advanced Food Research, Copenhagen, Denmark.

in western diets, most of them appearing as the simple carbs that should be avoided or enjoyed in moderation. A GI of 70 or above is considered high.

The cast of regular high glycemic foods includes most soft drinks, sports drinks, white bread, white rice, processed breakfast cereals, potatoes and watermelon. Even some otherwise healthy foods such as parsnips and dates can tip the scale with a GI of 97 and 103, respectively. Eat too many high glycemic foods quickly and you'll get the popular sugar high for up to an hour as blood glucose levels soar. Then comes the sugar crash -- the nappy, weak-kneed feeling that means your blood sugar levels have dropped to a level even below the starting point of the cycle. Plenty of enjoyable foods fall into the low GI (55 or less) and middle GI (56-69) strata, and not always where you expect. Black bean soup and a Mars bar share a Glycemic Index of 64, but not much else. Oat bran and a fruit cocktail share a GI of about 55. A serving of asparagus, artichoke or peanuts each has a GI of about 15. Skim milk and peanut M&Ms have a 32 GI in common, but little else.

If any fiber-rich food has a GI of zero, I haven't run across it. Ocean sand, perhaps, or wood chips? Make mine a shaved apple wood with a sprig of maple.

New studies are confirming the conventional wisdom:

High GI foods are making us soft.

A study at Children's Hospital Boston showed that junk carbs can spur a hefty increase in body fat, even without a gain in overall weight. Two teams of volunteer mice ate all they wanted for 18 weeks. Nutrients were the same, except one group got sugary carbs and the others a complex starch.

Although body weights remained equal, mice on the high GI diet had almost twice the body fat of the low GI mice after just nine weeks. After 18 weeks, the mice eating simple carbs "felt squishy" all over. When the experiment was terminated (along with the mice) researchers found the liver weights in both groups were identical, but the junk carb mice had 12 percent fat in their livers, twice the amount in the other group. Among humans, just 10 percent liver fat is considered an advanced stage of nonalcoholic fatty-liver disease.[130]

130: Janet Raloff. "Fattening Carbs -- Some Promote Obesity and Worse." Undated blog, *www. sciencenews.org*. The referenced study with mice was published in the August 28, 2004 issue of *Lancet* as: "Effects of Dietary Glycaemic Index on Adiposity, Glucose Homeostasis, and Plasma Lipids in Animals" by D.B. Pawlak and J.A. Kushner.

A somewhat similar study in Italy put 247 men and women into one of four groups based on their normal carbohydrate habits. Participants in the highest of the four GI groupings were found to be twice as likely to have undiagnosed fatty-liver issues.[131]

BREAD AND BUTTER

The message getting lost is that "if you reduce saturated fat and replace it with high glycemic-index carbohydrates, you may not only *not* get benefits, you might actually produce harm," says David Ludwig. He is director of an obesity program at Children's Hospital Boston. The next time you encounter a piece of buttered toast, he told Scientific American magazine, consider that "butter is actually the more healthful component." [132]

Good fats and complex carbohydrates are equally important to health, but not substitutes for each other.

It's like surfing. Or riding a bike.

Or stepping into a pair of tight sweatpants.

Balance matters.

131: Silvia Valtuena and others. "Dietary Glycemic Index and Liver Steatosis." *American Journal of Clinical Nutrition*. 2006.
132: Valtuena.

11

FAT FOOD POLITICS

When the U.S. Department of Agriculture was formed in 1862, it's mission was primarily to ensure a sufficient, reliable food supply and to disseminate useful information. The latter evolved into a mandate to issue sound dietary advice. As agriculture productivity improved by leaps and bounds, food producers turned to marketing to further increase profits. Harmony generally reigned through the 1960s, when government was still mobilized to fight its "war on hunger" among the nation's young, old, and poor. Within a few years, that battle was largely won.

"Eat More" was a message that producers of grains, meats, oils and dairy products could get solidly behind.

But "Eat Less?"

By 1969, producers were facing a new battle, one where nutrition was about quality, not quantity, and the concept of "bad" foods was taking hold. That was the year a White House Conference on Food, Nutrition and Health dared to suggest we eat less of the "unwise" foods containing too much sugar, fat, cholesterol and salt. Emboldened by a flood of studies blaming the American diet for increases in coronary diseases, a federal committee in 1977 recommended we eat *more* fruits, vegetables, whole grains, fish, poultry and nonfat milk, while eating *less* meat, eggs, fatty foods, sugar and salt.

The "Eat Less" recommendations "generated nothing less than an uproar," according to Marion Nestle, an influential nutrition researcher and policy watchdog. "Cattle ranchers, egg producers, sugar producers, and the dairy industry registered strong protest at the very idea that Congress might be telling the public that their products were bad for health."[133] And just like the tobacco interests who lobbied for a "sensible" emphasis on economics over health concerns, food producers and their farm state elected officials mobilized to protect their interests.

The politicized give-and-take on nutritional advice has continued ever since. Conservatives argue correctly that the public should be free to choose from the legally produced foods available to them. Progressives argue convincingly that objective recommendations regarding nutrition and prevention of disease are fundamental to promoting public health and controlling medical expenditures.

Along the way, food producers learned new rules of the game, reformulating, repackaging and "fortifying" a bajillion foods and drinks to tout exaggerated health benefits faster than the Food and Drug Administration was able to police the claims.

The wrangling never stopped, of course. The Congressional mandate to review nutrition guidelines every five years gave opponents time to come up with new studies and arguments. All the while, agriculture interests were free to promote their products in ways that would become thoroughly ingrained in public consciousness.

"Beef. It's What's for Dinner."™

"Pork. The Other White Meat."™

"Got Milk?" ™

"Lard: The Lube You Love."

Okay, that last one didn't catch on, but only because there was no Lard Producers Check-Off program to create an American Lard Institute to mount a big Lard Lovers advertising campaign. In the pseudo-reality of Washington, nutritionists and food producers kept returning to the impact of certain descriptor words to go with cautions about fats, sugars and salt. Words and phrases such as "choose," "go easy on" and "limit your intake" were dissected,

---

133: Marion Nestle. *Food Politics: How the Food Industry Influences Nutrition and Health*. Los Angeles: University of California Press, 2002

accepted or rejected. Advisory committees made up of nutritionists and industry representatives continue to thrash out every syllable of every recommendation about healthier eating.

Still, the 2005 overhaul was a big step in the right direction. For the first time, the USDA recognized most Americans were well-fed and then some. The overarching message paired calorie consumption with exercise to improve weight control. Anyone with web access and a little determination found ample information.

But the revisions also replaced the venerable food guide pyramid and its clear foundation of grains, fruits and vegetables topped by lesser amounts of proteins, dairy, fats and sweets. As a graphic, the new MyPyramid was merely a colorful, confusing splash of triangles and spilled groceries. Critics faulted the USDA for caving in to industry pressures by failing, once again, to clearly communicate what to eat less of. "In the final version, the USDA eliminated all traces of hierarchy," according to Nestle, "presumably because food companies do not want federal agencies to advise eating less of their products, useful as such recommendations might be to an overweight public."[134] It also meant that a growing number of health and elected officials were buying into the industry mantra of "balance, variety and moderation." Dietary advice, like the global warming debate heating up alongside, was pitting hard science against personal beliefs and opinions.

TOUGH LOVE

Jump forward to 2010 -- a five-year span during which the predominant health headline in the news related to an alarming development that was always termed "the obesity crisis." The reports were usually accompanied by stock photos or video of headless fat children and adults with the shameless moxie to be seen out of doors in full daylight and enjoying a waddle along public sidewalks.

While not directly acknowledging that news media had pushed an elephant into its conference room, the 2010 Dietary Guidelines Advisory Committee immediately recognized that, on the basis of the vast amount of newly published

---

134: Marion Nestle. "Eating Made Simple." *Scientific American*, September 2007.

research on obesity and its causes, a candid, updated report was needed. For the first time, the guidelines committee said it was addressing an American public "of whom the majority are overweight or obese, yet undernourished in several key nutrients."

The new guidelines dug in with tough love: "On average, Americans of all ages consume too few vegetables, fruits, high-fiber whole grains, low-fat milk and milk products, and seafood." That "Eat More" advice was followed up with some long-awaited "Eat Less" wording: Americans, they had discovered, "eat too much added sugars, solid fats, refined grains and sodium." Solid fats and added sugars (SoFAS) alone account for about 35 percent of calories in the American diet. Getting off the SoFAS, the committee said, "can lead to a badly needed reduction in energy intake and inclusion of more healthful foods into the total diet."[135]

The 2010 update also abandoned 2005's feel-good concept of "discretionary calories." The committee apparently recognized that adhering to its healthy food recommendation was challenging enough without a daily allowance for candy bars and caramel lattes. Although lacking any rule making authority to actually enforce its recommendations, the advisory group also criticized the overall "food environment" and called for beefed-up nutrition and physical education in schools. Families, it said, also need to work on their cooking skills, learning how to actually prepare and consume healthy foods at home.

Finally! A committee reporting to the USDA had delivered a veiled apology to fluffy and guilt-ridden Americans, conceding that overweight and obesity are not merely a matter of personal responsibility, but a societal problem requiring broad-based solutions. At last, "we look beyond wagging fingers and saying 'eat more fruits and vegetables,'" said consumer activist Marge G. Wooten, "and look at barriers and call for a national strategy to help people follow the recommendations."[136]

Various sectors of the food industry immediately responded to the new guidelines, calling them smart or ill-informed, according to where they fell in

---

135: Nestle.

136: Denise Mann. "Proposed Dietary Guidelines Take Aim at Obesity" *WebMD Health News*. June 15, 2010. Marge G. Wooten, PhD, is nutrition policy director of the Center for Science in the Public Interest.

the Eat More/ Eat Less continuum. Meat producers whined about seafood getting top billing in the protein category. Beverage makers countered that they offer a wide range of calorie choices. Spokesmen for The Salt Institute (There really is one.) rolled their eyes and called the lower sodium recommendations drastic and unrealistic. Fruit and vegetable producers liked the guidelines but their migrant workforce was too tired or undocumented to celebrate.

MyPLATE

Of course, it will be a cold day in Key Largo before many Americans read anything longer than a tweet before deciding what's for supper. Six months after restoring its credibility with its much-improved set of dietary guidelines, the USDA unveiled the federal government's new food icon. The confusing, reviled and embarrassing MyPyramid had been replaced with something to easily remind Americans to base each meal around a nutritionally balanced plate. It was, in fact, an image of a nutritionally balanced plate.

The graphic, called MyPlate, is divided into four nearly equal sections. The two largest are labeled for grains and vegetables, with two slightly smaller sections reserved for fruits and protein. To the side of the plate, a circle graphic grants permission for a serving of dairy -- presumably skim milk or low-fat yogurt, not pudding or a milkshake. A small field of accompanying text cut straight to the basics:

Enjoy your food, but eat less. Avoid oversized portions. Make half your plate fruits and vegetables. Make at least half your grains whole grains. Switch to lower-fat milk. Compare food labels for foods like soup, bread and frozen meals -- and choose the ones with less salt. Drink water instead of sugary drinks.

Wow! I'm impressed! Here, from an agency of the U.S. government, is a simple message and graphic, rich in information and void of fat and politics. Can bipartisanship, a comfortable bra, or a one-page telephone bill be in the near future? Nowhere on MyPlate is there a reminder to eat sugars, fats or carbs. That's not a prohibition -- just an acknowledgment that we'll surely find a way to include them. Likewise, the traditional "meat and beans" category is simply called "proteins" -- a suggestion that the nutrient is more important than the source, which could be seafood, tofu or any lean meat.

Nutritionists, in general, applauded the new graphic, especially those who had long recommended a return to the plate theme first used in the 1940s and again in the 1980s.

TOWARD A MORE SCIENTIFIC AMERICAN DIET

It took thousands of days, pages of recommendations, hundreds of comments, agile negotiations, and a few backroom deals. But finally, the lead health and agriculture agencies of the federal government served up their eighth edition of Dietary Guidelines for Americans. The 2015 blueprint gave dietitians and public health advocates reason to celebrate. It left enough wiggle room for profit-minded special interest groups to put on a brave face or even claim victory. Most of all, it was a political decision.

Sugar: The advisory committee shaping the eventual guidelines had recommended a tax on most sugar-sweetened beverages, as well as avoidance of artificial sweeteners. The final report didn't go that far. It agreed that sweetened soft drinks, sports drinks, and fruit drinks with less than 100 percent real juice can contribute extra calories "while providing few or no key nutrients." It sought to mitigate concerns about artificial sweeteners, saying that any sugar substitute in widespread use had already been approved as safe by the Food and Drug Administration.

For the first time, however, the guidelines were specific about the intake of added sugars, suggesting they account for no more than a tenth of daily calorie intake. On average, Americans now get 13 percent of daily calories from added sugar, with nearly half of that coming from sweetened beverages. Intake of added sugars is typically higher among children, teens and young adults.

As mild as the sugar warning was, the sugar industry challenged the science behind it, asserting in a statement that the committee had relied on "hand-picked science to support their predetermined conclusions."[137]

Ironic, much? Some nutritionists say the sugar industry has excelled at doing exactly that for decades.

Meats and fats: As always, meat producers were on the offensive while

---

137: "The Sugar Association Responds to 2015 Dietary Guidelines Advisory Committee Report." The Sugar Association web page statement. February 19, 2015.

the advisory committee was reviewing thousands of studies. Various beef, pork and meat "institutes" spent more than $1.1 million on lobbying in 2015, even launching an online petition for a "Hands Off My Hot Dog" campaign.[138] You didn't hear about that one? Perhaps they should have enlisted someone in the mold of the late actor and First Amendment advocate Charlton Heston. He could dare us to pry a steaming chili dog from his cold, dead hand.

The advisory committee had pressed for an explicit recommendation to limit the consumption of red meat and processed meat, which have been linked to heart disease and cancer. Instead, the final document takes the less offensive (to meat producers) approach of targeting nutrients. It recommends that no more than 10 percent of daily calories come from saturated fat, which is a natural component of red meat and many other tempting foods.

On average, Americans get 4.4 percent of their saturated fat intake from burgers and another 4.1 percent from other beef dishes. But give cheese credit for its contribution of 8.5 percent, and that's not including pizza -- 5.9 percent. Chicken dishes, dairy desserts and grain-based desserts each contribute 5.5 to 5.8 percent. Even reduced fat milks claims 3.9 percent of the average daily intake. That's according to the American Cancer Institute, which is officially unhappy the final guidelines gave a pass to eat red meat, as long as it is lean.

"There is strong evidence that red meat consumption increases risk of diabetes, heart attacks, stroke and some cancers (especially processed meat)," said Dr. Walter Willett, head of the nutrition department at the Harvard School of Public Health. "And there is not good evidence that this is simply due to the fat content."[139]

The guidelines continue to recommend low- and no-fat dairy products, despite recent studies indicating that whole milk may instead be the better choice for controlling weight.

Cholesterol: The 2015 guidelines take a broader approach to dietary cholesterol, removing the hard cap of 300 milligrams daily. Lately, research has

138: Helena Bottemiller Evich. "Meat Industry Wins Round in War Over Federal Nutrition Advice." www.politico.com. January 7, 2016.

139: Maggie Fox. "New Federal Dietary Guidelines Are Out, and No One is Happy." NBC News, as posted at www.wrcbtv.com. January 7, 2016.

reversed years of Conventional Wisdom which had linked the cholesterol we eat to the serum cholesterol in our blood. The American Egg Board (sounds official — and it is!) proclaimed a new era of freedom for its confused consumers, even though the long version of the guidelines says that dietary cholesterol is still an important consideration and should remain a minor component of a healthy eating pattern.

More important than focusing on dietary cholesterol or total fats in general, Americans should be most mindful of the saturated fats associated with most meats and dairy products. Remember, too, that many processed foods touting their "low-fat" attributes have actually increased the calorie count by adding even more sugar and simple carbohydrates.

Salt: The updated guidelines make only subtle changes in previous benchmarks and still suggest a limit of 2,300 mg per day for most people, while saying those predisposed or diagnosed with hypertension should shoot for 1,500 mg per day.

But have you heard? Studies completed in just the last few years have challenged the Conventional Wisdom by concluding there is no clear benefit to reducing sodium.[140]

One study which randomly assigned patients with congestive heart failure to either a low-sodium or normal diet was particularly surprising. Those put on the low-salt diets had significantly more hospital admissions during the study's follow-up period. When eight other trials involving more than 7,200 participants were analyzed, analysts found no reduction in all-cause mortality in the subgroup that had been following doctors orders to cut back on salt.

"I'm pretty immersed in the medical literature, and all of this is still shocking to me," wrote Aaron E. Carroll, who studies the studies for readers of the New York Times. "It's hard to overestimate the effect of the dietary guidelines. Hundreds of millions of people changed their diets based on these recommendations. They consumed less fat, they avoided cholesterol and reduced their intake of salt." [141]

140: Aaron E. Carroll. "Behind New Dietary Guidelines, Better Science." *Nytimes.com*. February 23, 2015
141: Carroll.

FIND FOOD. EAT IT.

Not only have some earlier major recommendations come to be viewed as unnecessary or unhealthy, a major consequence of the don't-eat-that warnings was to steer the always-hungry American diet toward more carbohydrates — especially sweeteners and nutrition-stripped grains — a trend that is only now becoming the mainstream explanation for the rise of obesity.

In the run-up to rewriting the 2020 dietary guidelines, the Salt Institute will no doubt be circulating the newer, salt-friendly science on Capitol Hill, just as lobbyists from The Sugar Association and American Bakers Association will seek to protect their industries from whatever carb critics are bringing to the debate.

Public health, profits, and politics will always compete for prominence in the dietary guidelines. Like our preference for thick burgers and watery beer, that's just the American way. But when meal times come around, true patriots should seek to honor the standards of theirs foremothers who managed to prepare healthy meals in tiny kitchens and a small inventory of vegetables, fruits, and wheat or corn.

Today, we're told to focus on what the experts call "nutrient-dense foods." Back in the day, without all the hyper-processed foods and drinks competing for shelf space and appetites, they just called it *food*.

PART TWO

TAKING CONTROL

12

INTUITIVE EATING

E xperience has taught most of us that the second day of a diet is easier than the first — usually because we're already off the diet. One notable exception was the Texas man who was ordered to begin a low-carb diet, shot his doctor, and then spent the rest of his life with only bread and water.[142]

Embracing the Fat Smart Happy lifestyle isn't a license to gain more weight or reason to keep from dropping a few pounds. Nor does it require losing weight as a precursor to happiness. In fact, that's just plain backwards. It's happiness that leads to weight loss.

So get happy! Start by eating whatever you want, whenever you want!

The fine print for this plan, which I'm including right here in a regular-sized font, is to *factor in healthy foods, reasonable portions, and enough sleep and activity to maximize your body's inborn power to take good care of itself.*

Come on. We're adults here. Do we really need another diet book, spouse, parent or cardiologist to tell us when we've had enough to eat?

I am reminded of the stomach-churning scene in the movie *Monty Python's The Meaning of Life*. If you saw it, you can't forget how the morbidly obese character Mr. Creosote is persuaded, after eating multiple portions of every item on a French restaurant's menu, to ingest a "wafer-thin" mint.

142: It's good that you're checking the footnotes. The incident cited here is almost certainly a complete fabrication.

This evidently was the tipping point, as graphically illustrated when the gourmand then literally explodes into a slurry of quail eggs, bechamel sauce, and entrails. Clearly, Mr. C's body was having its final say about the risks of gluttony.

And it's a vivid reminder to listen more carefully to the subtle cues your body provides long before reaching a life-threatening emergency.

What I'm advocating here is a non-diet approach which, in less opulent times, was merely described as eating. Today, to distance it from the fad and restrictive diets promoted ad nauseam, the discipline is referred to as *instinctive eating, normal eating,* or *conscious eating.* I think it would be helpful to simply call it *refueling,* or *replenishing,* which shifts the emphasis to why we really need to eat. But I'm okay with "Intuitive Eating," the nomenclature currently in vogue among authors and academia. It simply means relying almost completely on common sense and the grumbling noises in your stomach to tell you when you need to eat.

It's not a quick way to lose weight, by any means. But is can help lower your metabolic set point and make sustained weight loss easier. Many practitioners have found it a stress-free way to sample all their favorite foods while slowly losing healthy amounts of weight over a period of months and even years.

In time, intuitive eaters will settle in at their natural weights. The Battle of the Bulge just ends quietly and naturally with a cease-fire. That's it. It's over. No drama. Just a naturally-sized you. Peace at last. Hug yourself! Hug a tree! Skip and go naked! Go naked and (carefully) hug a tree!

Let's break it down to the ABCs. For our purposes here, A is for the new attitude that gets you started on the path to Intuitive Eating. B is for the behaviors you will embrace and practice to make it work. And C is for the cravings and contrarian thinking you will learn to deal with effectively. It might even stand for crazy, which is how your friends and family are going to react to your freedom and success.

ATTITUDE ADJUSTMENT

The previous chapters have provided ample and, I believe, persuasive information to form a durable foundation for your new attitudes about health, weight, and eating. We know that obesity is increasing globally. We know that being somewhat "overweight" actually predicts a longer life, while obesity requires extra effort to offset associated health risks.

We know that multi-billion dollar food producers, processors and marketers are motivated to provide you with a staggering supply of fats, sugars and other carbohydrates. We know that a massive weight-loss industry is selling little more than hope and dreams, and would go out of business if their products and services actually produced long-term results!

We know that our genetic predisposition to store fat and prepare for famine has been coddled and super-sized by an environment of cheap calories and push-button conveniences. We know that the safety and effectiveness of medical interventions have been compromised by profit-driven marketing and lax regulation. And we know that weight-loss dieting is an ineffective and often dangerous eating disorder.

Because dieting and guilt have become the new norm, we don't want to be normal. Our contrarian attitude is that *eating is normal*, and that individually, the best advice on what and when to eat comes from within.

Can you hear it? If not, close your eyes and stick a finger in your belly button. Seriously. Jiggle the contents a little and just listen to your stomach. And if you don't get a firm answer, move on to something else or just wait another 15 minutes to ask yourself: Am I really hungry? What kind of fuel exactly is my body hungry for?

This will take a week or so of practice. The challenge, of course, is to distinguish between legitimate hunger and the emotional eating habits you've developed over a lifetime. A bad day at the office or a broken heart can easily trigger emotional eating. So can good times, good friends and good food. Or a hundred other emotionally minor events, good or bad, which make up our daily life. Routines or habits with strong food associations occur throughout the day: An office meeting and a doughnut. The commute home and caramel latte. TV and Tostitos. Sex and sangria. Bedtime and cookies.

There are a thousand emotional reasons to stuff your face, but only one reason to fill your stomach. Be conscious of the lazy eating behaviors you have learned to ignore. Here's one of those little tips that is worth anywhere between zilch and a million dollars depending on how seriously you embrace it.

Write it down.

Just carry a little notebook or note-taking app and write down everything you eat and drink whether you are hungry or not. It's easier than counting calories, and you can eat whatever fits into the ol' pie hole. But within a week or two at most, you ought to feel more than a little lax if the daily lists aren't getting any shorter. Decide that it's easier to take a deep breath or a stick of gum than to write down gratuitous eating episodes. And when you're not hungry at all, make that grocery list of rewarding, healthy foods.

While developing a smarter, more deliberate attitude toward eating, begin making your peace with the lovable and huggable shape you see in the mirror. We'll talk more in a later chapter about society's fat phobias, but for now focus on your own attitude about fat acceptance. Remind yourself so that you can later remind others: Body size — thick or thin — does not reflect personal worth.

Before his rise and fall in the U.S. Senate, comedian and writer Al Franken was on Saturday Night Live poking fun at life coaches with his yellow-sweatered Stuart Smalley character. Well, just try reciting the Smalley creed in the mirror every day, and see if you don't start feeling better about yourself.

"I'm good enough. I'm smart enough. And doggone it, *people like me!*"

And if that's not digging deep enough into your psyche, just remember that Mr. Rogers likes you just the way you are.

So let's dump all of that complicated, perfectionist thinking. The unrealistic expectations of weight-loss dieting are a sure path to disappointment, guilt, and self-loathing. Get over your "all or nothing" attitude about what to eat today. The decision about whether you are hungry for celery or candy is yours to make. With Intuitive Eating, there are no good or bad days. They're all pretty good days; some just taste better than others.

You may not trust yourself just yet, but I do. Studies at Ohio State University have shown that college women given unconditional permission to eat do not binge and gain weight. They actually reached a lower weight than a group which did not follow Intuitive Eating principles. Related studies there also showed that intuitive eaters also were happier with their bodies, more optimistic, and better able to deal with stressful situations.

"Healthy eating is associated with psychological well-being in a lot of different ways," says Tracy Tylka, co-author of the studies. An individual's ability to listen to body signals and eat appropriately, she says, "seems amazing, but it is true." [143]

Too often, Tylka says, women believe that some degree of body dissatisfaction is healthy if it provides motivation to slim down. "But it may be just the opposite," the psychology professor says. "An appreciation of your body is needed to really adopt better eating habits."

Okay, but isn't a non-structured, non-diet really a license to binge and add pound? "That's not what we found," the researcher says. "If you listen to your body signals in determining what, when and how much to eat, you are not going to binge and you're going to eat appropriate amounts of nutrient-dense foods."[144]

Other studies at Ohio State found similar conflicts of self-image and health among men, especially those who want to achieve the lean and muscular look that media stereotypes equate with power and success. Tylka says there's a difference between men who exercise and watch their diet for their health and men who are focused on changes that pop out of a mirror. "They're not eating healthy," she says of gym rats determined to bulk up. "They are cutting out major food groups like carbohydrates and eating massive amounts of protein."[145]

EFF THE EFFING DIET

If this all seems too academic or hypothetical, consider the line of thinking adopted several years ago by the comedienne Margaret Cho. Not a woman inclined to skimp on the "F" word, Cho fell into something she calls, um, The "Eff It" Diet. After a period of rebellion against diets, small meals, no carbs, supplements and exercise, Cho decided to eat just what she wanted. She gained weight — for a while.

143: "Women Who Accept Their Bodies More Likely to Eat Healthy." News release from Ohio State University, August 8, 2006. The studies were presented at the annual meeting of the American Psychological Association.
144: Same as above.
145: "Pressure To Be More Muscular May Lead Men To Unhealthy Behaviors." News release from *Ohio State University*, August 10, 2006, coinciding with Psychology Professor Tracy Tylka's presentation at a meeting of the *American Psychological Association*.

"Then I started to get weirdly thinner," Cho explained in a blog. "I get it now. Because I don't care about food. It is there when I want it. I don't crave it and want it and think about it. Since I can have everything, nothing is that important. When I am hungry, I eat."[146]

And dimpled actress Melissa McCarthy. After a year or more of losing an estimated 75 pounds so gradually it nearly went unnoticed, McCarthy revealed her "secret" was simply the realization that stressing about her plus size was her real problem.

"I truly stopped worrying about it," McCarthy told a perplexed Gayle King on *CBS This Morning.* "I stopped over-analyzing, over-thinking, over-doing anything. I kinda went back to when I was pregnant and I just stopped constantly being worried about it and I think there's something to kinda loosening up and not being so nervous and rigid about it that, bizarrely, has worked. I could've figured that out before 44, but whatever."[147]

You can borrow Cho's name for an undiet if it suits your style, or come up with your own. The important thing is adopt some new behaviors to build on your new attitudes about dieting and self-acceptance.

BEHAVE, YA'LL

Perhaps the healthiest aisle in the grocery store is the one stocked with plastic wrap, freezer wrap, foil, resealable bags, hard plastic storage containers and garbage bags. Swing by the hardware aisle and pick up a decent microwave oven for the price of three pounds of crab claws. Then learn how to gently reheat those encore meals.

If cable TV can re-re-repeat *The Lord of the Rings* or *The Shawshank Redemption* twice a week forever, you can create some enthusiasm for one plate of leftovers. When eating out, push the excess away or ask for a carry-out box. There's no shame in getting two meals for the price of one. Your server sure doesn't care, so long as the tip is thoughtful.

I get that "Don't worry, be happy, eat smart" is easier said than done. So

---

146: margaretcho.com/blog/fuckitdiet. November 6, 2003.
147: Claire Rutter. "Melissa McCarthy Finally Reveals Her Weight Loss Secret After Dropping the Pounds." June 3, 2015. www.mirror.co.uk

let's break Intuitive Eating down to some baby steps, as compiled by dietitian, counselor and Olympic-qualified marathon runner Evelyn Tribole. Her 2012 book, *Intuitive Eating*, explains the philosophy and mechanics in hand-holding detail.

Here are some key principles (also available, and more, at the website *intuitiveeating.org*.)[148]: Reject the diet mentality: The best use of books and magazine articles promising fast and easy weight loss is for lining a litter box.

If you allow even one small hope to linger that a new and better diet might be lurking around the corner, it will prevent you from being free to discover Intuitive Eating, Tribole says.

Honor your hunger: Rebuild trust in your body's signals of hunger and satiety. Depriving yourself of needed energy and nutrients will lead to excessive hunger and loss of control.

Fire the food police. In the lawless world of Intuitive Eating, you are not the sheriff or a criminal depending on whether you follow or ignore your gut reactions to certain foods. It's better to enjoy a piece of fudge in the moment than to manufacture feelings of deprivation which lead to intense cravings, then binge-eating and guilt. When food rules are outlawed, there are no eating laws to break.

Respect fullness. It is defined by your stomach and satiety hormones, not by what is left to eat and how it tastes. Instead of eating quickly in an effort to clean the plate, take a breath. And another. Whether a food is simply delicious or just nourishing, give it the respect it deserves. Slow, mindful eating enhances the pleasure and satisfaction of eating. Yup, Intuitive Eating is sexy!

Keep foods and feelings separate. Mad? Sad? Bored? Lonely? Emotions deserve attention, but food won't solve the problem. "If anything, eating for an emotional hunger will only make you feel worse in the long run," Tribole says. Instead of solving one problem, overeating adds another layer of guilt and discomfort.

148: "10 Principles of Intuitive Eating." © 2013. *Intuitiveeating.com*. The website is a collaboration of Evelyn Tribole and Elyse Resch, nutritionists and eating disorder counselors based in Newport Beach, Calif. They also have a favorite food in common: dark chocolate, savored slowly.

Health matters. "Forget militant exercise. Just get active and feel the difference," the diet counselor says. Nor does making thoughtful food choices mean being perfect every day. "It's what you eat consistently over time that matters. Progress, not perfection, is what counts." [149]

149: "10 Principles of Intuitive Eating." © 2013. *Intuitiveeating.org*.

13

SCHOOLS, KIDS, FOOD AND FITNESS

What about the kids?

As the grown-ups in this room, we've taken a hard look at the forces, inside and out, that push and pull adults as they attempt to cross the balance beam of life without dropping their gym shorts. Adults make mistakes and are expected to make amends or live with the consequences. Fair enough.

But what about the kids?

Sure, they are maturing faster physically than they did in previous generations, but their first 10 years or so are still micro-managed by parents and educators. What to eat, where to attend school, what time to turn the lights out -- these parameters of daily routine are largely set by adults. Even imperfect or overweight parents can still impose rules with a "Do as I say, not as I do" immunity from fairness and reason.

Not many parents will brag over coffee or beers that they are doing their best to make sure their children are fatter than all their classmates. ("Yeah, Junior's fussy sometimes. But when I tell him he can't have a chocolate milkshake until he finishes his French fries, you'd be surprised how motivated he gets!")

But real encouragement to bulk up is often directed toward high school athletes, especially in wrestling or football, where college scholarships and even professional careers are bankable incentives. Two studies of more than 4,000 high school football linemen in Iowa and Michigan found that 45 percent of them were overweight, including 9 percent who would be considered severely obese as adults. We're talking about boys in the mid-teens weighing 300 pounds of more.

Their classmates on the chess and debate teams aren't doing much better.

One third of all kids ages 2 to 19 are fat by BMI standards. Fifteen percent of all kids are at least overweight; another 18.2 percent are full-on obese. That's 33.2 percent above the mainstream definition of normal. The boys are a little chunkier than the girls, 33 percent versus 30.4 of girls who are overweight or obese. Race, for whatever reason, also seems to be a factor. While "only" 15.2 percent of white youth are considered to be obese, 22.9 percent of Hispanic youth and 25.7 of blacks fall into the obese spectrum. Lumping all that lumpiness together, more than 41 percent of black and Hispanic youth are overweight or obese.[150]

If none of this is weighing heavily on parents, it's probably because adults are twice as likely to be eligible for fat camp. Estimated by BMI, 33.1 percent are overweight, another 35.7 percent are obese and 6.3 percent (more than one in 20 adults) have earned extreme obesity status with a BMI of 40 or higher.

It is an amazing but accepted deviation from statistical standards that every parent's child happens to be smarter and better looking than average. Decency dictates that the rare exception to this rule is charitably paired with the phrase, "Bless his/her heart."

So it was no surprise when a study showed that even though most parents agree childhood obesity is a major health issue, more than 40 percent of parents of clinically obese children ages 6 to 11 describe their progeny not as obese, but as "about the right weight." Less than 10 percent of parents of obese children in that age group said they are "very concerned" about their child's weight. Concern grew with age, however, with parents of kids ages 12 to 17 more than three times as likely to express their worries in that poll.[151]

150: "Overweight and Obesity Statistics." National Institute of Diabetes and Digestive and Kidney Disorders within the *National Institutes of Health*. www.niddk.nih.gov. The latest available figures in 2016 were for 2010.
151: "Poll: Kids' Obesity Not Weighing on Parents' Minds." News release, *University of Michigan Health System* for the C.S. Mott Children's Hospital National Poll on Children's Health and Knowledge Networks, Inc. December 10, 2007.

The least-concerned parents may assume their fat kids eventually will "grow out of it," although there is ample evidence that overweight at any age is the best predictor of increased overweight in the years ahead. Parents, regardless of their own weight, may also embrace the fallback position that good exercise and nutrition habits, like everything from ABCs to STDs, are best taught by professional educators. And why not? Schools have the gymnasiums, athletic fields and cafeterias. Where better to institutionalize the good habits that are being marginalized everywhere else?

SCHOOL SPENDING ON A DIET

Any school worth its opening bell wants to be part of the solution. But consider what's been heaped on their plates. Since at least the 1970s, schools have been pressured by state and federal legislators to do a better of job of preparing students to compete in a global, service, and high-tech economy. Good idea, although it required extra staff, focus, and funding.

Another mandate came with a 1972 amendment to federal education law. Title IX (Nine), as it was called, clearly prohibited sexual discrimination in any education program receiving federal funds, including physical education and athletic programs.

Also a good idea. Also very expensive to implement.

True gender equality in public schools required costly modifications or additions to locker rooms, equipment, playing fields and team sport offerings. To partly offset these costs, most public high schools would, over the next five years, eliminate physical education requirements for juniors and seniors. Local school boards could often rationalize that private fitness centers and soccer leagues were sprouting up to fill the void, at least for those who were affluent and motivated enough.

The new academic and fitness initiatives would have been an ambitious challenge even if school revenues were keeping pace. But taxpayers, especially the aging empty-nesters, were feeling squeezed too. Local school boards that refused to make quick spending cuts risked facing permanent caps dictated by public initiatives such as California's Proposition 13, a 1978 referendum. Passed by voters in a 2:1 margin, the amendment to the state constitution slashed property taxes — the primary source of school funding — by an average of 58 percent. Taxpayer-led revolts quickly spread to other states, and the impact is still being felt.

A great many positive trends in education had their origins in the Golden State. Even so, Proposition 13 set the table for unwelcome trends that would spread from coast to coast, border to border. Within two years of its passage, and even as enrollments were growing, the California Department of Education ended a program that had provided millions of dollars for the maintenance and upgrading of school cafeterias. Many schools, squeezed for space, turned to serving foods prepared off-site.

By the 1990s, fast food giants like Taco Bell and Pizza Hut — long resistant to freezing or reformulating their foods to meet lunchroom nutrition requirements — were being invited to set up carts in the hallways just outside the federally protected boundaries of the cafeterias. Within a few more years, a majority of California's public schools were subsidizing their cafeterias by offering branded foods, including pizza slices with twice the calories of the bland school pizzas covered by U.S. Department of Agriculture guidelines.[152] Oh, and the branded food was *making money* for the schools.

And what beverage goes best with a gooey slice of *as-seen-on-TV* pizza? Answer: Not milk. Some of us geezers fondly remember a lone vending machine outside of the school cafeteria which dispensed, for a nickel or a dime, a six-ounce cup of Coke. Today, or course, a 12-ounce can of soft drink is usually the smallest vending size available, and vended cans have been nearly eliminated in favor of "value-priced" 20-ounce plastic bottles.

A 1998 federal study confirmed the ebb and flow of drink habits. In just 12 years, milk purchases by schools fell 30 percent while orders for carbonated beverages jumped 1,100 percent. Later studies would draw other parallels between increased soft drink consumption and rising rates of childhood obesity, bone fractures and caffeine dependence.

School boards may have nodded in agreement when dentists and nutritionists stepped forward to label soft drinks as nothing more than liquid

---

152: Greg Critser. *Fat Land: How Americans Became the Fattest People in the World.* Boston: Mariner, 2003.

candy, but when it came time to hammer out a balanced budget, the generous offers from soft drink distributors were still ringing in their ears.

It's a poorly kept secret that soft drink giants have found room in their billion-dollar advertising and promotion budgets to reach children at an earlier age, even licensing the use of their logos for baby bottles. The goal is not just to quickly expand sales in the youngest demographics, but to jump-start brand loyalty for a lifetime of soft drink consumption. And where better to target those efforts than in a school's hallways, bus loading zones, and sports facilities?

Schools are typically able to stock their vending machines with soft drinks purchased in large quantities at half than retail prices. That standard mark-up to $1 or more per 20-ounce bottle can generate $25,000 a week for a district with 10,000 students. The deals are even more lucrative for the hundreds of districts which enter into exclusive "pouring rights" contracts with either Coke, Pepsi or Dr Pepper. Under these negotiated agreements, schools can hold out for large up-front payments, free drinks for sale in fundraisers and cash bonuses for reaching sales targets. Contracts may also ensure students are exposed to constant advertising reminders including soft drink logos on vending machines, cups, sportswear, brochures, scoreboards and even entire buildings. Lucrative? Enough so that many school districts employed experienced consultants to help them get the sweetest deals from the tooth decay fairies.[153]

KIDS FOR SALE

For nearly a century, well-intentioned federal health officials have attempted to promote sound nutrition in schools, only to butt heads with Congress and their generous campaign contributors in the snack foods industry. The give-and-take of the debate often focused on whether "foods of minimal nutritional value" (USDA-speak for junk food) should be allowed to compete directly with cafeteria foods without restrictions on the time and place of sale. In 1972, Congress tried to have it both ways by amending the 1996 Child Nutrition Act to permit the sale of competing foods during meal times — if the proceeds were used to benefit schools or school groups. In other words, it was okay to sell colas and corn chips if the Fitness Club got a few bucks out it.

153: Marion Nestle. *Food Politics: How the Food Industry Influences Nutrition and Health.* Los Angeles: *University of California Press, 2002.* See Chapter 9, "Pushing Soft Drinks."

Throughout the 1980s and 1990s, the U.S. Department of Agriculture, with support from nutritionists and school food service personnel, continued to press for restrictions on school sales of soft drinks and junk food. But soft drink producers, often with encouragement from school principals, funded strong legal challenges in the federal courts. Since the mid-1990s, Congress has shown the most resolve at the elementary school level by ordering firm limits on the sale of competing foods. Still, enforcement of federal guidelines has been virtually nonexistent, leaving state governments and local school boards to establish and enforce tougher rules on their own.[154] Some states have. More haven't.

THE PHYSICAL AND EMOTIONAL TOLL

Clearly, there are many school policy issues deserving front-burner attention at the local, state and national levels. But let's put any thought of possible solutions on a back burner long enough to reflect on why all of this is worth getting steamed up about. Parents who have successfully struggled to find their own path to fat acceptance have the same duty as any adult, thick or thin, to improve every kid's chance for a happy and healthy childhood. Health risks for children generally increase with the extent and duration of obesity. And we know the severe emotional damage heaped on heavy children can be harder to shed than the pounds which triggered their cycle of despair.

So we need to ask hard questions when the data miners tell us the number of young people who are overweight has tripled since 1980. We need to fidget when we drive by an empty playground on a Saturday. We need to do some soul-searching when we learn that barely half of kids today eat even one serving of a fruit or vegetable a day. (No, French fries don't count.) And we need to take action when many health professionals warn that childhood obesity may hasten the advent of Type 2 diabetes, asthma, high blood pressure, and heart disease.

Grow old and fat, and your knees hurt. For those who are fat, young and surrounded by schoolmates, the pain comes from frequent, emotional kicks in the gut. Children are adept at inflicting subtle cruelties, and physical differences are not well tolerated. Even though obesity is much more common, researchers say peer stigmatization is still prevalent and begins as early as age 3.

154: Nestle.

In a classic study first conducted in 1961, hundreds of 10- and 11-year olds were shown six drawings: a normal weight child, an overweight child and four others either in a wheelchair, on crutches, with an amputated hand or facial disfigurement. Asked to rank them in order of who they would want to be friends with, the fat kid was deemed least likable. When the study was repeated in 2003 with the same pictures, the fat child was again least popular, and by a wider margin.[155]

Another trio of researchers went so far as to compare the quality of life of an obese child with that of a child with cancer. Seriously? But it is true, researchers said, after objectively measuring the impact of their conditions in terms of school achievement and physical, psychological, social and emotional well being.[156]

"These kids are facing stigma from everywhere they look in society, whether it's media, school or home," says Rebecca M. Puhl (Ph.D) at Yale University's Rudd Center for Food Policy and Obesity.

Weight bias remains socially acceptable, is rarely challenged and often ignored, Puhl said after reviewing 40 years of related research.[157]

The analysis showed that kids who are bullied or teased because of weight are two to three times more likely to suffer from eating disorders or report suicidal thoughts — not surprising when parents and teachers (who should know better) often reinforce the biases voiced by children, or even sew the seeds of stigma themselves.

So who is responsible for broadcasting all that negativity in school? Well, at the risk of vilifying the vilifiers, just about everyone. The review by Yale researchers found that:

- Girls react more negatively to overweight classmates, even showing disdain for average weight peers.

155: Richardson, Goodman and others. (1961). "Cultural Uniformity in Reaction to Physical Disabilities." *American Sociological Review.* Also, Latner, J.D., & Stunkard, A.J. (2003). "Getting worse: The Stigmatization of Obese Children." *Obesity Research,* 11, 452–456.

156: Schwimmer, Burwinkle, Varni, (2003). "Health-Related Quality of Life of Severely Obese Children and Adolescents." *Journal of the American Medical Association.*

157: Associated Press article by John Christoffersen, published in several newspapers, including USA Today, July 12, 2007, under the headline "Overweight Kids Face Widespread Stigma." Puhl, the researcher quoted in the article, was lead author of the study, "Stigma, Obesity, and the Health of the Nation's Children," published in the July 2007 issue of *Psychology Bulletin.*

- Weight bias is evident among preschoolers, well-entrenched by the elementary level and doesn't reach a plateau until early adulthood.

- Caucasians exhibit the most weight bias; African American females are the most tolerant.

- Overweight and obese children of all ages are just as likely to hold negative attitudes and stereotypes about obesity as average weight children.

- Like adults, children who believe that weight is primarily a matter of personal control express the most negativity toward the overweight.

- One-fifth of educators believes obese persons are more emotional, less tidy and less likely to succeed.

- More than half of educators believe obesity is caused by a lack of self-control or compensation for a lack of love or attention. The greatest negativity is expressed by professionals who have made a career of fitness — physical education teachers.

The avenue of anxiety which connects obesity with low self-esteem is a two-way street, especially for children. Not only can weight issues trigger depression and absenteeism but, as another recent study showed, teen girls who placed themselves below average on a school's social ladder gained, on average, 11 pounds more than their more confident classmates over a two-year period.[158]

BACK TO THE RANCH

There's no denying that the school environment plays an important role in shaping the physical and mental health of kids all across the BMI spectrum. Many local schools, with or without help from the state and federal government, have invested heavily in time and money to push special nutrition education programs.

Some interventions are as simple as exposing youngsters to new foods, as public health officials did during a visit to a Baltimore-area elementary school. Some second-graders found something to like in the sweet slices of honeydew

---

158: Tara Parker-Pope. "School Popularity Affects Girls' Weights." *well.blogs.nytimes.com*. January 9, 2008.

melon and kiwi, but slices of green peppers and zucchini were a harder sell. One eight-year old screwed up her eyes at the vegetables, and then slurped down the small bowl of Ranch dressing which had been offered with them for dipping.[159]

And so it goes across the country. School districts that make healthier foods a part of their regular lunchroom offerings are learning that apples and celery don't make dollars and sense. In North Carolina, schools tried replacing a la carte items such as French fries and fruit-flavored drinks with real fruit and juices. Food costs went up. Sales went down. Within a five-year period, a statewide child nutrition program with a profit of $5.6 million wilted into a loss of $5.7 million.[160]

Dozens of other school-wide interventions have been attempted, including federal subsidies to provide free fruits and vegetables and offering prizes to kids who picked the most of healthy options. And usually it's the Ranch dressing that gets the best response. The Associated Press reviewed a stack of scientific studies that closely examined the outcomes of 57 special school nutrition education programs and "found mostly failure. Just four showed any real success in changing the way kids eat."[161]

Researchers reported kids were developing more positive attitudes about healthy foods as a result of the nutrition programs, but weren't actually changing their eating habits. The analysis cited the same counter-influences prevalent away from school — disinterested parents, money issues and relentless marketing of unhealthy foods.

British researchers came to similar conclusions when they followed the results of a year-long "Ditch the Fizz" campaign to discourage children from partaking of soft drinks. Two years later, they found that kids in the program had gained slightly less weight than a comparison group with no intervention. But after three years, the difference was nil. [162] Another British study refuted a parliament proposal to routinely screen all primary school children so that overweight and obese children could be offered special treatment. Why weigh

---

159: Ruma Kumar. "Giving Peas a Chance, Reluctantly." *Baltimore Sun*. March 23, 2008.
160: Michael Hewlett. "School Systems Losing Money on Stale Sales of Healthy Foods." *Winston-Salem Journal*. February, 23, 2008.
161: Martha Mendoza, Associated Press. "AP: Nutrition Education Ineffective." *USA Today*. October 25, 2007.
162: "Diet Education Had No Long Term Impact On Childhood Obesity." *www.sciencedaily.com* Posted October 9, 2007.

each child, the researchers asked, when there was so little evidence showing preventive approaches or treatments had any long term impact?[163]

TRY, TRY AGAIN

So why should any school eat up valuable time and limited resources with nutrition programs that have only a brief or modest chance of reversing obesity trends? Because — even though nutrition education programs have been scattershot and disappointing — schools "appear to be more a part of the solution than the problem." So says Douglas Downey, a sociology professor at Ohio State University, and co-author of a study that dared to compare days spent at school to days spent at home.

Compared to the months kindergarten was in session, BMI rates for children grew more than three times faster during their summer vacation. Among first-graders, the lazy days of summer saw BMI increases that were double what occurred while school was in session.

Obese children benefited the most during school months. That's when their rate of BMI gain was slowest, compared to other weight groups. Conversely, kids who were underweight tended to move toward a healthier weight while school was in session.

It all makes sense, the researchers concluded, because schools provide kids with a structured environment with limitations and expectations about what foods are served and when. (The same goes for adults who eat less during the work week than on weekends.) Schools can help kids by providing healthier food choices during schools hours. But the biggest contributors to childhood obesity will still occur outside of school, says Paul von Hippel, also a co-author of the above study. Schools can help by teaching children how to make healthier food choices all the time, in or away from school.[164]

163: "Doubt Cast on Routine Screening to Pick Up Overweight and Obese Schoolchildren." *British Medical Journal* news release, April 20, 2007, via www.newswise.com.

.

164: Jeff Grabmeier. "Schools Help Hold the Line Against Childhood Obesity." Ohio State University news release, February 24, 2007. The study appeared that month in the *American Journal of Public Health*.

SEDENTARY EDUCATION

Most schools have to give themselves a failing grade for not providing regular access to physical education programs. Budget restrictions are still at play while responding to federal mandates to test, test, test for academic achievement.

Here's a new way to define ridiculousness. In 30 of these United States, some middle and high school students can earn required credits in physical education through *online P.E. courses.* Some actually have a real exercise component, but monitoring may be open to deception. ("Honest, Coach, the dog ate my fitness tracker.")

According to an American Heart Association review of related studies, many youths are increasingly sedentary throughout their day, meeting neither physical education nor national physical activity recommendations. Physical education in schools has been decreasing in recent years, the group says. Now only 3.8 percent of elementary schools, 7.9 percent of middle schools, and 2.1 percent of high schools provide daily physical education or its equivalent for the entire school year.[165]

Instead of waiting for a foundation grant or an hour in the school gymnasium, some elementary schools teachers are experimenting with physical fun *during* class time. Their kids are mingling jumping jacks and jogging-in-place with geometry, music and spelling. They are embracing innovative, low-cost programs originating in the private sector. Instead of taking time away from academics, they can blend brain time with dozens of brief exercises such as "Invisible Jump Rope" and "Conga Line Rhyme." Colorful incentives appropriate to the early grades are part of one package called *Take 10!* which includes activity cards, stickers and posters for tracking progress.

What if classrooms themselves were designed to promote exercise? (Thanks for asking. There are no flies on my attentive readers!) Prototype "chairless classrooms" are being fitted with podiums and standing desks. For sitting, chairs are replaced with large, colorful balance balls. Educators who've done their homework know that exercise and learning go hand in glove. Not

---

165: "Increasing and Improving Physical Education and Physical Activity in Schools: Benefits for Children's Health and Educational Outcomes." April 25, 2015 report by the *American Heart Association* and the *American Stroke Association.*

only does exercise help youngsters to burn calories and feel stronger, but studies also show a positive correlation between activity and better test scores.

POSITIVELY PARENTING

The same interwoven, positive attitudes about exercise also apply to educating children about nutrition. We know that kids who are chided about their weight or forced to eat healthy foods will stash Honey Buns in their book bags and leave their cafeteria's fresh fruits and vegetables for the waste bins. That's money down the Dumpster and more stigma, liberally seasoned with guilt and low self-esteem, heaped upon the picky eaters.

But a two-year experiment in Philadelphia showed how a school-wide, *positive* approach could reduce overweight by half. Without a big investment, school staff received nutrition education, then incorporated their findings into classroom routines, for example, by teaching fractions and geometry with pizza slices. What teachers did *not* talk about was fat and weight. Instead, healthy eating was promoted as a way to become *stronger*. The appeal to the fourth-, fifth- and sixth-graders in the study was immediate and persistent. "Nobody wants to stigmatize kids. Nobody wants them to feel bad about themselves," said one nutritionist involved in the study. "Focus on the positive and reward it." [166]

With a $5,000 community grant, an elementary school in Merced, California took an equally positive approach with its "Harvest of the Month" program. For one week each month, kids "celebrated" a new fruit or veggie, culminating in a "Try It Thursday." Students who tried the new foods earned stickers and qualified for contests and prizes. "You wouldn't believe what kids will do for a sticker," said the school's director of food services.[167] The stickers provide an immediate reward, and because they are naturally low in calories and high in fiber, certainly better than the coupons for free French fries at Mr. Burger that many schools once distributed.

I've run across numerous examples across the country and in my own backyard of parents making a big difference at the local level. Being a member of

---

166: Sandy Sherman, EdD, director of nutrition education at The Food Trust, a Philadelphia nonprofit group involved in the study, as quoted in "Schools Can Help Kids Win Weight Battle," by Miranda Hitti, *WebMD Medical News*, April 7, 2008.

167: Terri Soares, as quoted in "Healthy Choices a Success at Ada Givens (Elementary School)," *Knight Ridder/Tribune Business News*. Feb. 12, 2008, as published at www.schoolnutrition.org.

the local school board is an honor in most communities, and rare is the member who can't be persuaded to support improved foods and fitness for students, especially when parents, teachers and administrators present a united front.

In my native western Kentucky, creative partnerships made all the difference in making fitness affordable and available to all students. At one elementary school in a low-income neighborhood, the parent-teacher organization came up with $18,000 to build a quarter-mile asphalt walking track behind the schools. Soon, about a fourth of the student body was showing up *voluntarily* a half-hour before the first bell to walk or run laps.

Students in the junior and senior high grades of the city school as well as the surrounding county school district were provided ready access to modern fitness equipment, made possible in part by a contribution from the city's only hospital.

Then, about the same time the state was ready to impose rules for school vending machines, the district launched its own "Healthy Student and Staff Initiative." A planning committee of administrators, teachers, coaches and students joined with nutritionists, psychologists, and a nurse to make recommendations. There was push back from vendors and even some teachers who were used to passing out goodies and celebrating every birthday.

But snack rules were agreed to and celebrations trimmed to one a month. Students were invited to participate in taste tests to help select healthier lunchroom options they would actually eat. And they did. The percentage of high school students eating the federally reimbursed, higher nutrition lunches rose to 73 percent, up from 66 percent when French fries were really fried, not baked. And now nearly a third of students in all grades get out of bed a little earlier in order to have a good breakfast at school.

SAVE THE CHILDREN

Here is the headline which accurately captured the essence of a newspaper opinion piece by the provocative British media personality Janet Street-Porter.

"Let Adult Fatties Eat Themselves To Death.

The Kids We Can Save."

In the column, Street-Porter ridicules government programs in the U.S. and Britain which offer cash or vouchers to overweight adults as an incentive to lose weight. The author goes on to blame adult obesity on "willful self-abuse," which I certainly don't agree with. But I find her callousness less contemptible when she says, "It would be better to abandon the current generation of fatties and pour all resources into ensuring that the next ones grow up to be fit." [168]

Who can argue that adults have an obligation to teach their children, not only about the world, words and numbers, but also about nutrition and fitness? With a majority of adults in denial about their own children's weight issues, schools are a logical place to teach those lessons, especially with input from parents and support from private partnerships. Surely, ounces of early prevention will cost society millions less than the inevitable pounds of treatment.

168: Janet Street-Porter, Editor-At-Large, "Let Adult Fatties Eat Themselves to Death. The Kids We Can Save.," *The Independent* (U.K.), January 27, 2008.

14

RISH MANAGEMENT

Alife without risks would be bland indeed.

A calculated risk, whether taken on a whim or after careful reasoning, can be all it takes to discover a favorite new musician or writer, or to pucker up for a life-changing kiss, launch a new career or bury a bad relationship. A risk worth taking is one where the potential outcome is better than the status quo.

According to Conventional Wisdom, being overweight or obese is inherently a risky behavior, with the odds clearly stacked against your health and longevity. According to the standard line quoted by many researchers and medical specialists, being overweight "leads to" or "contributes to" asthma, Alzheimer's, diabetes, cancer, cardiovascular disease, kidney disease, osteoporosis, sexual disorders, complicated pregnancies and a shortened lifespan. The journals of epidemiology are stuffed tighter than sweatpants in January with CW conclusions that Weight A is "associated with" Disease B, or that Weight C "preceded" the onset of Disease D. And yet other, equally qualified experts say the hard evidence of direct causal relationships is scattered, often contradictory or weakly isolated from other likely contributors.

I was going to save the following point as the dramatic conclusion of this chapter, but it will be more useful for you to keep it in mind as we look individually at various "obesity related diseases." Here it is:

Regardless of an individual's Body Mass Index — thin, middle or heavy

-- the best course of prevention, or a major component of treatment, will be the same: Healthier eating and more movement. Not a Cinnabon and a nap. Healthy food and getting off the couch. Not exotic herbals or a trip to a Central American clinic. Better eating habits and long walks. Not gaining more weight in order to qualify for insurance coverage of gastric bypass surgery. Saying "Yes" to fresh fruits, vegetables and lean protein. Not "light" cigarettes and a pig's heart transplant. Keeping a journal of what you eat. Buying a $20 pedometer and a $40 set of dumbbells. Joining a friendly support group.

Ooh! Have you seen the modern, full-featured jumping ropes? Now they come with custom handles, swivels and ball bearings, a choice of rope materials, colors, adjustable lengths, jump counters and a carrying pouch. Super nice! But I have jumped right off this page. So . . .

Regardless of age, gender or size, the proper defense against disease is the same. *The same!*

It's smart, mindful eating.

It's any physical activity you can enjoy often. And if you happen to drop a few pounds, improve your muscle-to-fat ratio or feel better while fighting what ails you, you'll just have to learn to like your new thinner, stronger self.

DIABETES

The headline on a report widely circulated by the HealthDay News service read "Obesity Driving Diabetes Epidemic." In it, the lead author of a study by the U.S. Centers for Disease Control says the findings "certainly help make the case that obesity is a major factor" in the increasing prevalence of Type 2 (adult-onset) diabetes.

Indeed, the data shows the greatest increase in diabetes has been among those with a BMI of 30 and above. But the study is based on self-reported surveys, and partly reflects recent changes in diagnostic criteria for diabetes. Nothing in the study actually points to obesity "driving" a diabetes epidemic.[169]

In fact, other researchers more suspicious of Conventional Wisdom

---

169: Linda S. Geiss, MA et al. "Changes in Incidence of Diabetes in U.S. Adults, 1997-2003." *American Journal of Preventive Medicine.* 2006.

believe obesity and diabetes follow two parallel but separate paths. Glenn A. Gaesser, PhD, the Arizona State University fitness expert who authored *Big Fat Lies*, reminds us that diet and exercise, not BMI, deserve the most attention. "It is possible to greatly improve or even 'cure' diabetes and other serious health problems," Gaesser says, "while still remaining markedly overweight."[170]

Another recent study helped isolate the impact of obesity and diabetes on health. Diabetes is a strong predictor of acute organ failure and early death for the obese as well as the non-obese, even more so than the presence of obesity without disease, according to a study of more than 15,000 adults. BMI levels alone did not predict organ failure, investigators found. Still, diabetics had a threefold higher rate of organ failure compared to non-diabetics.[171]

Some experts already believe that as much as half of an individual's predisposition to insulin-resistance and Type 2 diabetes is purely genetic, and not simply a result of weight gain. In fact, insulin resistance may be related to the "thrifty gene" which prepares us for famine by contributing to weight gain.

Other research shows that insulin resistance appears *before* the onset of weight gain. Regardless, insulin resistance and weight gain become part of the same cycle where higher insulin levels promote weight gain and the extra fat increases insulin resistance, and so on, round and round. It's a repeating cycle that can become a death spiral.

Better eating and increased activity may not eliminate the extra weight, but it will diminish problems with blood sugar, hypertension and most other diseases "associated with" obesity.

HEART DISEASE

The "obvious" connections between obesity and diseases of the heart and cardiovascular system also have been challenged by Gaesser and others suspicious of profit-influenced alarmism from within the Obesity Industry.

You've often heard that excess weight "makes the heart work too hard" — yet all other forms of exercise are said to strengthen the heart and improve

---

170: Glenn A. Gaesser, Ph.D. *Big Fat Lies*. New York: *Fawcett Columbine*, 1996
171: Katarina Slynkova, and others. "The Role of Body Mass Index and Diabetes in the Development of Acute Organ Failure and Subsequent Mortality in an Observational Cohort." *Critical Care*. 2006.

circulation. Blood pressure is a measure of two factors — the strength of the heart pumping the blood and the resistance of the vascular system through which it flows. The CW assumes that obese people are more likely to have higher resistance to blood flow because of atherosclerosis — the accumulation of fatty deposits in the arteries and the eventual "hardening" of those arteries.

The contrarian view was well documented by Dr. William Bennett and Joel Gurin in their groundbreaking 1982 book, "The Dieter's Dilemma"[172] and again by Gaesser in 1996. Together they reviewed dozens of studies including several based on tens of thousands of autopsies. Smoking, high blood pressure and untreated diabetes were indeed factors in heart disease, they found, but not obesity alone. Newer studies done with X-ray and angiographic dye showed similar results, according to Gaesser. A 1991 University of Tennessee study of 4,500 older men and women, he says, even suggested the obesity was actually a protection against clogged arteries.[173]

A French study a few years ago may have come closest to putting the various contributors to heart disease in proper perspective. The team tracked the health of nearly 140,000 men and 104,000 women who had routine health checkups, including testing for high blood pressure, cholesterol and fasting glucose levels. Within the group, which was monitored over an average of 14 years, 42 percent of men and 25 percent of women were classified as overweight or obese.

The finding: Just being overweight is not a risk factor for heart disease. Add high blood pressure to overweight, however, and the risk more than doubles. For those with overweight, high blood pressure and high cholesterol, the risk rose to about 2.6 times normal. Diabetes alone, however, only caused a minor increase in risk. "The important message in our study," said team leader Athanases Benetos, M.D., "is that we observed that cardiovascular risk is not clearly increased unless hypertension is present in these overweight and obese subjects."[174]

A separate 2012 study of 22,000 middle-aged participants over seven years

172: William Bennett,, M.D. and Joel Gurin. *The Dieter's Dilemma: Eating Less and Weighing More.* New York: *Basic Books,* Inc., 1982
173: WB Applegate,, et al. "Case-controlled Study of Coronary Heart Disease Risk Factors in the Elderly." *Journal of Clinical Epidemiology.* (1991) 44:409-15.
174: Peggy Peck. "It's High Blood Pressure That Triggers Heart Disease in Obese." *MedPage Today.* September 14, 2005. The study cited appeared in the September 13, 2005 issue of *Hypertension, Journal of the American Heart Association.*

concluded that obesity, whether measured by BMI or waist circumference, was much less a factor in heart disease and death than general metabolic health risk factors as measured by markers such as blood pressure, blood sugar, blood cholesterol and inflammation. "People with good metabolic health are not at risk of future heart disease — even if they are obese," according to Mark Hamer, a lead researcher at University College London.[175]

If you don't believe that, you'll probably believe this one -- a contradictory study released just a few months later by Copenhagen University Hospital.

This one had more than 71,000 participants and concluded that among participants *without* metabolic syndrome, being overweight added 26 percent to the risk of heart disease and heart attack. For the obese, the risk factor jumped 88 percent. Authors of this study said the more favorable outcomes in other studies may reflect differences in weight among participants when they first entered the study group.[176]

Regardless of the role of overweight and obesity, there is ample evidence that diet (equally with genetics) affects cholesterol levels. High blood cholesterol is tied to high blood pressure and hypertension contributes to heart disease. It's never too early to be mindful of cholesterol, especially now that the American Academy of Pediatrics has reluctantly recommended that cholesterol-reducing statin drugs be prescribed for children as young as eight years.

Adults, meanwhile should ask their physician if a daily regimen of aspirin is appropriate. In one study group, aspirin was credited with a one-third reduction in heart attacks, although increased risk of gastrointestinal bleeding has to be considered individually. And there is at least one small study which showed an herbal remedy — grape seed extract — is effective in reducing blood pressure.

About half of Americans routinely use dietary vitamins and supplements. In the U.S., the bare-bones federal effort to evaluate safety and effectiveness or to regulate sales is evidence of sustained and powerful industry lobbying. With more than $20 billion in annual sales, there are ample resources to assist lawmakers with their non-stop re-election fundraising.

175: Aparna Narayanan. "Obesity Not Always Tied to Higher Heart Risk: Study." *Reuters Health* as included at news.yahoo.com. May 24, 2012.

176: Elizabeth Devita Raeburn.. "Excess Weight Hikes Cardiac Risk All On Its Own." *Medpagetoday. com*. November 11, 2013.

I certainly have not done enough research to opine in any responsible way. However, the University of Toronto, Ontario very recently published its "meta-analysis" of 179 randomized controlled trials relevant to supplements and cardiovascular disease. The findings warrant at least a brief mention here. Among the research team's conclusions:

- Vitamin B complexes, and folic acid in particular, been found to *reduce* the risk of stroke among regular users. And that concludes the "plus" column.

- Niacin and antioxidants appear to increase the risk of mortality.

- Vitamins A, B6 and E, multivitamin supplements, beta carotene, selenium, magnesium, iron, and zinc supplements had no significant effect on heart disease or mortality from all causes.

"In the absence of further studies," said Valentin Fuster, M.D., editor-in-chief of the medical journal which published the research, "the current data on supplement use reinforces advice to focus on healthy dietary patterns with an increased proportion of plant foods . . ."

There it is again. Real food, whole foods, are the best source of necessary vitamins and minerals, and a whole lot more.

Even so, high cholesterol, blood pressure, and blood sugar are all serious medical issues which may require additional treatment, often with inexpensive, time-tested, generic prescription medicines.[177]

CANCER

Cancer. The word alone conjures up horrific images, especially for those who have witnessed the misery of a loved one undergoing chemotherapy and radiation treatments, only to delay by a few months the painful and life-sapping power of mutating body cells. Yet, millions of lives have been spared by advances in cancer treatment, and many more potential cancers averted by generations of public education, especially about the consequences of smoking. A few years

---

177: Megan Brooks. Medscape.com. "Most Vitamin, Mineral Supplements Don't Reduce CVD." June 4, 2018. The study cited, "Supplemental Vitamins and Minerals for CVD Prevention and Treatment," was published in *Journal of the American College of Cardiology*. June 2018.

into this new century, statisticians were able to report for the first time a decline in the number of cancer deaths. Because of better screening and treatments, five-year survival rates for cancers of the colon, breast, blood, skin, prostate and pancreas all improved at the turn of the century, compared to 20 years earlier.

And yet the new villain in town — obesity — threatens to reverse that progress, according to a spate of new research. Bummer.

Obesity is just one of many potential contributors to cancers under continuous study by the National Institutes of Health's National Cancer Institute and private organizations such as the American Cancer Society.

The NIH review of 2007 data for the United States concluded that 34,000 new cases of cancer among men (4 percent of the total) and 50,500 women (7 percent) were "due to" obesity. It's not clear if the NIH chose those particular words in its 2012 fact sheet to declare a *causal* relationship between obesity and cancer. Elsewhere in the same document, cancer is simply "associated with" obesity in all but a few references.[178]

Specifically, the NIH says obesity is associated with increased risks of the following types of cancer: esophagus, pancreas, colon and rectum, breast (after menopause), endometrium (lining of the uterus), kidney, thyroid and gallbladder ("and possibly others as well.")

Any association between body weight and cancer is likely related to one or more of these specific factors identified by the NIH:

Fat tissue produces excess amounts of estrogen, high levels of which have been associated with the risk of breast, endometrial, and some other cancers.

Obese people often have increased levels of insulin and insulin-like growth factor-1 (IGF-1) in their blood which may promote the development of certain tumors.

Obese people often have chronic low-level inflammation, which has been associated with increased cancer risk.[179]

178: "Obesity and Cancer Risk." *NIH National Cancer Institute. www.cancer.gov.* As reviewed or revised January 3, 2012.

179: "Obesity and Cancer Risk." *NIH National Cancer Institute.* www.cancer.gov. As reviewed or revised January 3, 2012.

Fat, Smart, Happy risk managers want to know: Does losing weight lower the risk of cancer? The NCI says that for ethical and other reasons, there have been no large controlled clinical trials to answer that question. Back in 2004, the health agency said flatly there was insufficient evidence that intentional weight loss would affect the risk for any cancer. Its position was that even though some studies had suggested there may be a slight benefit, most of them had not adequately isolated whether an individual's weight loss was intentional or related to other health problems. (And, as noted earlier in this exquisitely sourced book, simply being underweight or of "normal" weight may be a drag on longevity.)

Today, the NIH says the same limitations to well-controlled studies still exist, but the federal research center and information clearinghouse mentions that a few observational studies have found decreased risks for breast cancer and colon cancer among people who have lost weight. Stronger evidence, it says, comes from studies of patients with an average weight loss of 30 percent following bariatric surgery. Those patients "appear to have lower rates of obesity-related cancers" than obese patients who bypass the bypass surgery. Surgery, of course, comes with its own set of risks.

SMOKING

Any useful advice about cancer, health and weight management presumes you are not a smoker. That's an increasingly safe assumption given the percentage of American adults who smoke has dropped from a peak of 42 percent in the mid-1950s to barely 15 percent today.

Public health officials long described smoking as the nation's leading cause of "preventable illness," contributing to 480,000 deaths annually. Now obesity holds the dishonor. Here's the little x/y chart version: In 1990, the declining line representing smoking prevalence criss-crossed with the uptrending line representing obesity rates. Since then, experts have said that obesity is the most significant drag on life expectancy.

We've talked at length about contradictions in the health and weight debate. But there is no disputing smoking's negative influence on heart disease and diabetes.

Nearly 41.5 percent of adults are either obese *or* smokers, but less than 5 percent -- about 9 million thrill-seekers in all -- are obese *and* smoking. [180]

Healthwise, it's a bad combination. Obesity and smoking combined can increase the risk of early death by two to six times, especially from cancer and cardiovascular disease. The combination is especially dangerous for women. [181]

Smoking is expensive and now on a par socially with drunk-dialing and leprosy, largely because of heavy taxes and the public education campaigns which have so effectively undermined the tobacco industry's subtle marketing and blatant lies.

Cruel ironies abound. For many smokers, cigarettes are fairly effective as an appetite suppressant. Smokers who manage to quit often gain five to 20 pounds within five years, potentially offsetting some health benefits.

Considerations will vary widely among individuals according to income, health and weight. Or just ask yourself which tastes better: a long drag on a cigarette named for a camel or a bowl of Moose Tracks ice cream?

ARTHRITIS

The most obvious correlation between weight and arthritis is best explained with the physics of gravity, motion, and friction. Even normal weight puts a steady pressure on all weight-bearing joints, especially the hips and knees. Injury, age, and heredity factor in as well, but weight takes the cake for wearing down the flexible cartilage that covers the end of bones where they are joined together.

One in five Americans has been diagnosed with arthritis. Among the obese population, that ratio jumps to one in three. Here's some more math. The experts have determined, somehow, that every pound of extra weight exerts the equivalent of another four pounds of pressure on the knees. So 20 extra pounds of weight is another 80 pounds of pressure on those joints. Fifty pounds becomes another 200 pounds squishing through your hips, knees and feet.

180: Cheryl G. Healton, and others. "Smoking, Obesity and Their Co-Occurrence in the United States: Cross Sectional Analysis." *BMJ.* July 1, 2006.

181: Peggy Peck. "Obesity and Smoking: A Mortal Duo." *medpagetoday.com.* October 3, 2006.

Little-known tip: Attaching yourself to a 1,500 cubic foot balloon filled with helium will lighten your overall load by 100 pounds while quickly diverting attention to your mental health.

Regardless of whether obesity contributes directly to arthritis -- or if the discomfort and inactivity characteristic of arthritis leads to obesity -- the weight of evidence suggests that in terms of personal comfort and mobility, weight matters.

One 2014 study blamed overweight and obesity for about 95 percent of the undisputed spike in orthopedic surgical procedures. From 1993 to 2009, the number of hip replacement surgeries in the U.S. *doubled*, according to the study, while the number of total knee replacements *tripled*. [182] The greatest increase in surgeries was among the same age group growing the most in girth, the 18 t0 64 year olds.

The spurt is all the more significant given the traditional reluctance of surgeons to perform hip or knee repairs until obese patients demonstrate their resolve with some significant weight loss. Extra weight may contribute to higher complication rates, post-surgery. Perversely, maintaining pre-surgery weight loss is more difficult for patients whose mobility is limited by pain in their hips and knees.

But a growing number of orthopedic specialists are looking beyond arbitrary cut-off points tied to height and weight measurements. And now there's a study to back them up. "Our evidence showed that severe morbidly obese patients can benefit almost equally as normal patients in pain relief and gains in physical function," said Wenjun Li, PhD. He is an associate professor of medicine at University of Massachusetts Medical School and lead author of a study involving 5,000 hip or knee replacement patients. [183]

"Patients who can lose weight should, but we acknowledge many people can't, or it will take a long time during which their joints will worsen," said Dr. Li. "If they can get the surgery earlier, once function is restored they can better address obesity."

182: Kiernan, Meghann. "Increase in Knee Replacement Surgeries Directly Linked to Obesity." *outsourcestrategies.com*. May 22, 2015. The referenced study appeared in the June 2014 edition of *Journal of Bone and Joint Surgery*.
183: "Study Finds Obese Patients Don't Need To Lose Weight Before Total Joint Replacement." News release. UMassMed.edu. July 19, 2017. The study cited was published the same day in the *Journal of Bone and Joint Surgery*.

As when considering weight loss surgery, would-be patients need to conduct adequate research and look for surgeons or practices which have performed hundreds of successful procedures.

KIDNEY DISEASE

High blood pressure and diabetes have long been associated with kidney disease, including the end-stage renal failure that requires a kidney transplant or, as 400,000 Americans are currently enduring, regular dialysis treatments. Only recently have researchers attempted to isolate the impact of obesity, apart from hypertension and diabetes. Two large, independent studies conducted in the U.S. and Sweden reached the same conclusion: Obesity, and even minor overweight, is a major risk factor.

Researchers at the University of California, San Francisco reviewed the files of 320,000 customers of a larger insurance company, including 1,471 who experienced kidney failure over a period of 26 years. Crunching the BMI numbers, they found the rate of failure among those who were merely overweight (BMI 25-30) was 1.87 times greater compared to those under BMI 25. And for the morbidly obese (BMI 40+), the occurrences of kidney failure were *seven* times greater, probably a result of kidneys working overtime to filter the larger amounts of blood.[184] Separately, a Swedish study evaluated 926 patients with moderately severe chronic renal failure. Focusing on age and gender as well, those researchers reported that risks were tripled for both men and women who were above BMI 25 at age 20 or later.[185]

I'm sorry I can't sugarcoat this kidney business a little for you, but it would take enough sucrose to send you into a diabetic coma. So you may want to skip the following factoid: If your kidneys are ready for the garbage pail but you're on the official waiting list to get a transplant, you may experience one final act of discrimination. Even where local physicians and hospitals declare that obesity is not a consideration in the fair allocation of donated organs, the reality is that the chances of receiving a kidney transplant are 27 percent less for patients in

---

184: "UCSF Study Finds Obesity a Risk Factor in Kidney Failure." News release, January 02, 2006, University of California, San Francisco. The study cited appeared in the January 3, 2006 issue of Annals of Internal Medicine.

185: "Obesity Triples the Risk of Chronic Kidney Failure." Newswise, May 11, 2006. The study cited, "Obesity and Risk of Chronic Renal Failure," appeared in the June 2006 issue of the *Journal of the American Society of Nephrology.*

the U.S. who are classified as severely obese (BMI 35-40), and 44 percent less for the morbidly obese. Although specialists say there is strong evidence that obese patients can benefit significantly from a kidney transplant, obese patients tend to have worse outcomes.[186] This, in turn, may affect a hospital's quality ratings – and insurance reimbur$ement$.

BRAIN DRAIN

As mentioned previously, advances in the treatment of heart disease, cancer and diabetes are allowing millions of senior citizens to live long enough to experience more "senior moments." Whether described as cognitive decline, dementia or Alzheimer's disease, the continuing loss of brain tissue brings on a heartbreaking endgame for the victims and their caregivers. Some researchers, thwarted in their attempts to find a cure for this natural downside of the aging process, have instead chosen to look for a new villain and believe they've found one in obesity.

In the last few years, various studies in the U.S. and Sweden have found *associations* between obesity and the loss of brain tissue or memory skills. But no causal relation has been identified, except to associate obesity with diabetes and hypertension – two conditions which may contribute to cognitive decline. It's also interesting to note that among women, but not men, unintentional weight loss begins about 10 years before the diagnosis of dementia. Women, it seems, may forget about preparing meals, but men rarely forget to eat. My layman's, men-are-from-Mars opinion on all this is as follows: If you are filled with dread about becoming so old you lose your mind, don't worry so much about trying to outlive diabetes, cancer, hypertension and other pre-emptive diseases.

PREGNANCY

Here, risk management means erring on the side of safety for both mother and child. This is why: An analysis of 54,000 pregnant Norwegian women found the risk of fetal death – or stillbirth, generally defined as the death of a fetus after 20 to 28 weeks of gestation – was double for overweight women (BMI 25-30) and more than triple when BMI was above 30. Let's say the real-world percentages are only half what the study concluded. That is still a big added risk.

186: "Extreme Obesity Affects Chances of Kidney Transplantation." *Newswise*, January 10, 2008. The study referenced was conducted by the Johns Hopkins University School of Medicine and published in the February 2008 *Journal of the American Society of Nephrology*.

Also, an Australian study tracked 14,000 women and found that high BMI was associated with higher rates of babies being born with birth defects, respiratory distress and hypoglycemia. A U.S. study said infants born to obese mothers had twice the chance of having one of seven specific birth defects including spina bifida, heart defects and missing toes, fingers or limbs.

Obesity is hard on pregnant moms as well. They are more likely to deliver prematurely, require caesarean section, and develop gestational diabetes or hypertension. And hard labor is longer, averaging 7.5 hours for overweight women and 7.9 hours for obese women, versus 6.2 for middleweights. Even so, experienced mothers who would do anything to trim an hour off the labor clock should not launch a crash diet after becoming pregnant. Sound nutrition is important to both mother and child during pregnancy. Instead, physicians say, mothers-to-be need to focus on healthy eating long before conception. Ladies, if you can navigate an Instagram feed, program your DVR to record *Dietland*, or find your way home from a tanning spa, you're smart enough to plan a safe pregnancy. Worldly men have been known to say the three best things in life are "a drink before and a cigarette afterwards" – wink, wink. Obese men hoping to become fathers may need to cut back on smoking, drinking and overeating because all three can contribute to infertility. However, the science here is quite muddled. Being overweight or underweight is associated with reduced sperm counts and concentrations, according to a study of 1,600 young Danish men. Another study involving 1,468 U.S. farmers and their wives suggested that a 20-pound increase in men's weight may raise their chance of infertility by about 10 percent.

Conversely, researchers at an English fertility clinic found no disparity in sperm quality across four different BMI groupings. And the most recent study, involving 300 very overweight men in New York, also found they were *not* more likely to be infertile. "We see pretty significant deficits in fertility in women due to obesity, so we thought we'd see an effect in men," the study's co-author said. "But that wasn't the case." [187]

187: "Overweight Does Not Decrease Sperm Production." June 15, 2008 news release from *The Endoctrine Society*, as reported by *Newswise*.

SHORT NEEDLES, LONGER STAYS

Overall, obese adults can expect to have slightly more hospital admissions -- 3.22 over 20 years, compared to 2.47 stays for "normal" weight adults, according to a Purdue University Study. Obese adults also will stay hospitalized a little longer (10.96 days compared to 9.4. days, according to the same study). The severely obese also will face the usual prejudices and some new indignities –syringe needles too short to reach the meat of the buttocks, blurry x-rays, cramped wheelchairs, aggravated MRI claustrophobia, or medical misdiagnosis.

A "ticking time bomb." That's how researchers in England described the impact of obesity and an aging population on national health care systems when they released the results of a study published in 2008. Increasing BMI correlated with a greater risk of physical impairment in men and women ages 65 and older, they concluded after tracking the health of 3,800 seniors.

The same study inadvertently confirmed a major factor in extra weight's role in disability: The overweight and obese oldsters also *lived longer*! Sure enough, the principal finding was that "participants in higher BMI categories had greater risk of impaired physical function at follow-up but little or no greater risk of mortality."[188] In fact, mortality rates for the overweight and obese were lower than for the "normal" BMI group with BMI 20 to 25. Only the severely obese (BMI 35+) were more likely to die during the study period.

Few people are blessed with perfect health and a natural, sudden death after completing a lengthy retirement bucket list. But fat, happy and guilt-free adults with a responsible approach to a healthy diet and appropriate exercise will not be denied their chance at longevity on the basis of weight alone.

All of the above health-related concerns are worth a frank discussion with your doctor and family, especially if you are very obese, have any of the related symptoms or precursors of a dangerous condition, or a family history of any disease. If your doctor's first reaction is "Lose 50 pounds and then we'll talk," you'll need to re-educate him or her regarding the new truths about weight and fitness, or shop around for a doc who has already embraced a more pragmatic, holistic approach to health. Even then, the physician's recommendation will

---

188: Charles Bankhead. "Obesity-Related Impairment in Older Adults Called Ticking Time Bomb." *MedPage Today,* August 26, 2008. The referenced study by Iain A. Lang, Ph.D., et al, was published in the August 2008 issue of the *Journal of the American Geriatrics Society.*

likely involve healthier eating, more exercise and a carefully considered and dosed prescription drug.

There may indeed be a strong case for weight loss – the kind that can often be achieved slowly, even permanently, through intuitive and mindful eating habits.

But if months or years of attempting a healthier lifestyle haven't sufficiently reduced your risks of serious illness or injury, it may be time to consider – long and hard – the most radical Rx of them all. Some activists for fat acceptance say there is never a strong case for weight loss surgery. I say . . .

15

WEIGHT LOSS SURGERY

Have you ever invited friends or relatives to your home for a formal visit primarily so that you have a firm deadline to clean house and clear the junk out of the guest room? The guys who wrote that *Freakonomics* book call that a commitment device. Perhaps the earliest such physical gimmick was a chastity belt, a crude but effective tool to restrict the free trade of any woman tested by open borders.

In each of the last several years, about 200,000 Americans signed a stack of liability waivers and said goodbye forever to Big Macs and breakfast buffets. What they got in return, at a cost of close to $40,000, was a surgically reconfigured stomach and/or colon that limited all future meals to portions about the size of a typical crash diet. The gastric bypass, adjustable gastric band, vertical sleeve gastrectomy and other variations of bariatric surgery have joined the hysterectomy and vasectomy as modern medicine's most accepted and life-changing commitment devices.

After a year of adjusting to the surgery and learning the hard way that greasy foods and sweets will cause sudden "dumping" trips to the bathroom, most patients are able to *slowly* ingest three small meals and an evening snack each day. A typical recommended dinner might include 3 ounces of grilled tuna, 1/2 cup of couscous, a smear of diet margarine and 1/2 cup of broccoli. After an evening snack consisting of 1 ounce of low-fat cheese and half a peeled apple, the mini-stomach will be ready the next morning for a down-home country breakfast. Translation: a cup of low-fat sugar-free yogurt and half a banana, sliced thin to discourage wolfing.

Obviously, a person who ate like this every day could shed just as much weight without undergoing a costly, potentially dangerous and certainly life-altering surgery. But "could" and "would" are two different things, especially for those who have tried and failed at weight loss for years. That's why traditional and newer versions of bariatric surgery have become the commitment device of choice for thousands of dangerously obese adults and even a few teenagers.

What's involved in the procedure? What are the benefits and concerns? What are the costs? Who's going to pay for it? Is it right for you? Will I quit teasing you with questions and provide some useful information already?

LONG STORY, SHORTENED

Surgical attempts to short-circuit digestion date back to the 1950s. But the procedures didn't go mainstream until they became the poorly kept weight-loss secrets of public figures such as Carnie Wilson, Al Roker, Randy Jackson, Rosie O'Donnell, Sharon Osbourne and New Jersey Gov. Chris Christie. Increasing obesity rates, more liberal attitudes by insurers and the advent of heavily promoted bariatric clinics have quickly elevated weight loss surgery into a billion dollar a year segment of the Obesity Industry that is certain to prosper for years to come.

You are well familiar with most aspects of the digestive process, starting with the most pleasant part -- the chewing and tasting -- and ending with the, uh, conclusion part. A normal stomach can hold about three pints of food at one time. That's where strong acids begin to break down the foods. Absorption of nutrients continues as foods wend their way through nearly 20 feet of small intestine. (Note to self: Ascertain if this is where Bose got the idea to fold a long sound baffle into their little speaker cabinets.)

In the first years of the bariatric boom, the most common procedure was the Roux-en-Y gastric bypass. I assume the name was derived from French recipes for chitlins.

No? Regardless, the procedure was a combination of tricks to restrict food intake and the absorption of some nutrients. After a lot of anesthesia, snips, and stitches, the patient is left with a smaller stomach pouch, combined with a bypass around most of the stomach and small intestine to reduce caloric intake.

It is highly effective. Most patients shed 65-70 percent of excess body weight after one year. A commitment device of the first order, the Roux-en-Y gastric bypass is almost always irreversible. The undoing is costly, risky, and more complicated than the doing.

There had to be a better way.

The less-invasive adjustable gastric band has become the less-is-more alternative. Gastric banding works primarily by decreasing food intake. Surgeons are able to use the less-invasive laparoscopic technique, making small poke- and peep-holes in the lower abdomen to install a silicone bracelet around the upper part of the stomach. A valve stem left implanted just under the skin allows doctors to make slight adjustments to the circumference of the inflatable silicone ring. You probably should not ask for a weekend special just to pig out during Thanksgiving.

Weight loss with gastric banding is slower than with bypass surgeries, but results are about the same after three years. Advocates say the risk of surgical complications and nutritional deficiencies is lower with banding. Recovery is faster. Scarring is minimal.

But as more patients were logging more years with the gastric bands, shortcomings came into focus. One study found the bands had eroded in one of three patients, and that 60 percent required additional surgeries. Another study showed half of patients with bands needed additional surgeries to make adjustments or deal with complications.[189]

But supporters of banding say the dominant complication is financial and procedural. In Australia, where follow-up care is covered by national insurance, Paul O'Brien, MD, a pioneer in the Lap-Band® method, says the initial surgery is only the first step. "There are plenty of people out there doing this surgery without a follow-up program for their patients," he told WebMD's Laura J. Martin. "And they are setting them up for failure."[190]

In the U.S., where even the initial surgery is not always covered by insurance, some surgeons are backing away from gastric banding. The percentage of weight

---

189: Laura J. Martin, MD, reviewer. "Lap-Band® Shown Effective for Long-Term Weight Loss." Webmd. com. January 18, 2013.

190: Martin.

loss surgeries at Lenox Hill Hospital in New York involving gastric banding dropped from 40 percent to about 3 percent from 2009 to 2012, according to Martin's reporting. An official at Vanderbilt University Medical Center in Nashville told her that just five of the 360 weight loss surgeries done there in 2012 used the Lap-Band®. "We have essentially stopped doing this operation," said Ronald H. Clements, MD, head of the university's bariatric surgery program. "The sleeve and the bypass are just better for helping people lose weight and keep it off. That's what we are seeing in our patients and that's what the data are telling us."[191]

A spokesman for the trade group representing most bariatric surgeons agreed the banding procedures requires regular maintenance and adjustment. But it's still a good option for many patients who choose surgeons with a policy of scheduling regular follow-ups, he said.[192]

The "sleeve," referenced above, is an up-and-coming technique, properly called the vertical sleeve gastrectomy. It is performed via laparoscopy and involves removing part of the stomach and using staples to create a smaller tube-shaped stomach. Advocates say the method is safer because it doesn't leave any foreign materials to cause complications. It allows the stomach and intestines to function normally, reducing the chance of poor nutrition intake associated with gastric bypass surgery, while still encouraging weight loss.

Meanwhile, surgeons and their suppliers are looking at new alternatives. For the most extremely obese patients, it may be possible to reduce the risk of medical complications by performing surgery in stages, first using a less invasive procedure to bring weight down to a surgically safer level then returning months later for a more complicated bypass. Simple, non-surgical remedies continue to draw interest, along with questions about safety and effectiveness. It's very simple to use oral endoscopy to insert one or more balloons into the stomach to take up space and curb appetite, usually for a period up to six months. Experience will determine if the method is too simple

---

191: Martin.
192: Martin. The statement was from James Ponce, MD, president of the *American Society for Metabolic & Bariatric Surgery*.

HOW FAT IS FAT ENOUGH?

Barely 7 percent of bariatric surgeries are performed on patients who cover all costs out of their own pockets. That gives insurance companies and regulators the biggest voice in deciding who qualifies for a surgical intervention. Although surgical specialists and their equipment manufacturers are already lobbying for more lenient criteria, the standard set by the National Institutes of Health has been to limit surgery to those who are severely or "morbidly obese." That ominous classification means a BMI of at least 40 or, for examples, 270 pounds for a man of average height (5 feet, 9 inches) or 230 pounds for a woman (5 feet, 4 inches.)

Actually, that's the standard for an individual who is both "morbidly obese" and fairly healthy. The accepted standard for surgery drops to a BMI of 35 in the presence of certain "comorbid conditions" including diabetes, hypertension, sleep apnea, gastric reflux, osteoarthritis and diseases of the gallbladder, liver, and cardiovascular system. Throw in a diagnosis or two of lower back pain, herniated disc, deep venous thrombosis, infertility, urinary incontinence or cataracts and you'll have an even more compelling argument for getting surgery approved. In 2011, the FDA also approved two methods of gastric banding for adults with comorbidities and BMI as low as 30.

More than 220,000 Americans undergo weight-loss surgery each year, according to the American Society for Metabolic & Bariatric Surgery. Yet that was only a tiny sliver of the tens of millions in the adult population that would be considered eligible for a procedure.

Four out of five people undergoing weight loss surgery are women -- probably because they experience more discrimination in relationships and the workplace. The average age of people going under the bariatric knife has been increasing and is now in the early 40s. The vast majority occur in the 35-54 demographic, but the fastest growth is among those 50 and over. Physicians and insurers are increasingly willing to approve weight loss surgery for the 60-and-over crowd now that studies have shown they get the same benefits and have a rate of postoperative complications comparable to younger people. Also increasing is the number of bariatric patients under age 20 and as young as 12 -- mostly females dogged by depression and comorbidities. The only diminishing aspect seems to be the stigma attached to the surgery itself.

Even so, candidates will have to do more than meet weight and complication requirements. A competent surgeon is also going to involve a team comprising your family doctor, a psychologist, a dietitian and other professionals in a pre-screening process designed to identify hidden medical problems and fairly calculate the ratio of benefits to risks.

A good medical team will screen patients thoroughly in advance to identify emotional problems and evaluate each candidate's chances for success. Insurance companies will also demand their pound of justification. Some will insist on documentation showing that legitimate efforts to lose weight through dieting and other non-surgical methods have failed.

LESS YOU, MORE HEALTH?

Strictly in terms of weight loss, the benefits of surgery are well documented by now. After just one year, those receiving a full gastric bypass can expect to lose up to 80 percent of excess weight while a drop of 40-50 percent is considered normal with gastric banding. Weight loss continues for 18 to 24 months, then levels off. And yes, some weight gain is expected again between two and five years after surgery. Simply because of the weight loss, most patients report an improvement in their moods.

Nothing wrong with that, but your doctors (and insurance company) are more impressed with the collateral improvements in health. High blood pressure is corrected in about 70 percent of patients, sufficient to reduce or eliminate medications and cut the risk of coronary-related deaths by half. An excess of fatty lipids is corrected in about 70 percent of patients. Sleep apnea and the snoring that goes with it are eliminated within a year for most patients. Type 2 diabetes is reversed in the great majority of patients. Often, blood sugar levels are normal within weeks of the surgery, even cutting the eventual cause of death due to diabetes by 92 percent.

Still, there are legitimate debates about whether the long term benefits outweigh the short-term risks of surgery, including infections, and the lifelong compromises imposed by a commitment device.

Remember, maintaining weight loss is going to require all the same sacrifices that make dieting such a chore. Smaller meals, healthier snacks and calorie-cutting are part of the package. Willpower still matters. Even a stomach one-fifth its original size can accommodate a large Rocky Road milkshake a few sips at a time.

Sticking to the new dietary requirements can take months to accept fully. For some, depression sets in and won't let go, sometimes ending in suicide. And for as many as one in four patients, the forced end to out-of-control eating is regrettably resurrected as an "addiction transfer." Denied self-destructive eating habits, the still-troubled patient turns to drugs, alcohol, gambling or even compulsive shopping.

For most patients, sanity and energy return about three months after the surgery.

UMM, WHO'S GOING TO PAY FOR THIS?

Employers are becoming more willing to pay for weight-loss surgery as they collect data predicting their eventual savings or "payback" by avoiding other health care costs associated with obesity. Even so, only a small percentage of those eligible for surgery at little or no cost to themselves are willing to undergo a procedure, regardless of their current weight and health concerns.

Since 2006, the federal Medicaid assistance program for lower-income adults has paid for all major flavors of bariatric surgery for "morbidly obese" candidates with at least one serious comorbidity such as hypertension, artery disease, or osteoarthritis. In 2008, Medicaid wisely extended its criteria to include Type 2 diabetes. Medicaid only covers procedures performed within high-volume, "high-quality" facilities as recognized by the American College of Surgeons or the American Society for Bariatric Surgery.

During one three-year period, nearly 75 percent of all procedures were covered by commercial insurance. Combined, Medicare and Medicaid paid for another 15 percent.[193]

All patients, regardless of who's footing the bill, should insist on the same credentials. Detailed information about patient outcomes at nearly 700

193: Carol Nicholas and Rick May. *HealthGrades Fifth Annual Bariatric Surgery Trends in American Hospitals Study.* Health Grades, Inc., Golden, Colorado. May 2010.

hospitals and surgery centers is available from HealthGrades, an independent ratings organization. The group even has a "Five-Star Rating" for hospitals with the best history of patient outcomes.

BUT IS IT FOR YOU?

Nothing says commitment (or desperation) as convincingly as turning your personal weight management over to a stranger with a face mask and sharp knives.

Clearly, comorbidities, costs, and complications are all legitimate concerns for any elective surgery. But studies, averages, advocacy groups, insurance companies and books like this are just the information starting point for anyone seeking to strike the proper balance of caution and courage.

For the heaviest patients with clear evidence of weight-related health problems, the first question may be "Why do I keep putting this off?" But all candidates for surgery need to devote months to gathering facts, having candid discussions with family and friends, exploring online forums and dropping in on local support groups for post-surgery patients.

Successful candidates will also have to undertake an objective self-analysis to look for deeper, unresolved issues that can't be fixed by sutures and staples alone.

16

HEALTH IN ALL SIZES

Recall, please, two very important truths lavishly documented and earnestly reported in previous chapters. One: Weight is an unreliable, even deceptive indicator of an individual's physical health and personal worth. Two: Eating and exercise habits primarily directed at losing weight rarely succeed beyond a few months while inflaming and prolonging negative consequences. Frequent weight-loss dieting easily morphs into an entry-level eating disorder marked by poor nutrition, energy loss, weight gain, increased frustration and lowered self-esteem.

Any list of the most vulgar, demeaning four-letter words in popular parlance has to include d-i-e-t. Agreed? There is an alternative, one that has been gaining popular support and academic credibility. One version has become so clearly defined its founders registered for a trademark. It's called Health At Every Size®. Or HAES®.

So, yes, there is a sensible alternative to sacrificing health and self-esteem in the vain and dangerous pursuit of weight loss. It is an emphasis on health without the emphasis on weight. The formula is the same dog-eared recipe for health that's always made more sense than money: smarter eating, more physical movement, less risky behavior. If, to you, this lacks the freshness and excitement of front-row tickets to see Metallica, Beyonce, or the Super Bowl, stimulate your cerebrum with this review of the folly of weight-centered dieting.

Genes rule. Your body's inherited characteristics include powerful instructions to gain weight in preparation for a famine that may never come. Genetics influence the hormones which signal hunger and fullness. Your body has powerful metabolic safeguards to maintain and defend a weight that is natural to you. That natural weight, or set point, increases with age.

Dieting is a disorder. Anorexia, binge eating, and weight-centered dieting all have the same unhealthy relationship with food. Each psychopathy is characterized by an intense fear of gaining weight, exaggerated influence of weight on self-image and obsessive categorization of foods as either good or bad. Diets don't work. Weight loss is almost always temporary. Deprived of calories, the body makes adjustments to maintain weight, and the pounds come back. Losing weight can shorten your life. Losing the same few pounds over and over again (weight cycling, or "yo-yo" dieting) is especially unhealthy.

As obvious as it must now seem to my enlightened readers, it only took a millennia or so for mankind and womankind to learn, then forget, then rediscover the truths about healthy eating. First, there was that long phase where populations were primarily motivated by the belief that it was better to eat than be eaten. As civilization flourished, the next health goal of the masses was to become as fat as the king. Well into the 1800s, heftiness and health were considered synonymous from birth. In 1876 America, when having a "fine fat baby" was still every mother's goal, popular artist John Rogers sold thousands of copies of a 120-pound sculpture called "Weighing the Baby." In the carving, the baby has been nestled in the grocer's desktop scales while an older brother is seen tugging down on the baby's blanket -- to increase its weight. [194]

Then, as farm subsidies and agriculture science pushed the cost of producing a calorie to near zero, stockholders and advertisers insisted that every value-added one of them find an open mouth. And it came to pass that obesity settled on the land as if a host of locusts had transformed into French fries and gummy bears. Rather than attack the source with something as simple as larger nutrition labels and smaller cola cups, policymakers took the mantle of kings. Now that fat had trickled down to the lower classes, they declared it was ugly, contemptuous, and dangerous. Fat is for fatheads. Thin is in. Simple as that.

194: Hillel Schwartz. *Never Satisfied: A Cultural History of Diets, Fantasies & Fat.* Anchor Books. Doubleday. New York. 1986.

To justify their contempt, the fatphobia fanatics only had to trot out the growing mound of research *associating* obesity with illness and disease. Most of that research, however, had skimped on proving an actual causal relationship. Mostly, the new findings were built upon the wobbly foundation of previous studies -- all of which were predispositioned, intentionally or not, to reach the same weight-biased conclusions. The few studies that dared to contradict the accepted narrative were hard to find and rarely acknowledged outside a core group of broad-minded academics.

Mercifully, this version of The Hungry Games has seen the emergence of a resistance movement. The uprising emerged armed to the teeth with a passion for social justice and unbiased science.

TERRORISTIC THREATENING

In 2005, Michigan State University nutritionist Jon Robison, PhD, joined forces with a dozen other nutritionists, researchers and authors to create the Health At Every Size journal. His editorial was a call to arms incited by no less than Richard Carmona, then surgeon general of the United States. "Obesity is the terror within," Carmona said during a public lecture in February 2006. "Unless we do something about it, the magnitude of the dilemma will dwarf 9/11 or any other terrorist attempt." [195]

Robison responded that the public had become confused and frightened about their own bodies and the food they eat because of the biased research and reporting, the profit-driven promotion of dangerous diets and surgeries, and the recent recommendation that children be given BMI report cards. "In the past few years, the hysteria over the 'obesity epidemic' has reached its own 'epidemic' proportions," Robison said. "Ironically, as in the past, the one result that is *least* likely to occur from the heightened hysteria for the vast majority of people is long-term weight reduction." [196]

Later that year, Robison and his contrarian colleagues were invited to elaborate on the tenets of Health at Every Size in a newsletter for the hundreds of

---

195: Jon Robison, PhD, MS. "Health At Every Size: Antidote for the 'Obesity Epidemic.'" *Health at Every Size* (the Journal). Volume 19, Number 1, Spring 2005.
196: Jon Robison, PhD, MS. "Weight, Health & Culture: An Historical Perspective." *Absolute Advantage*, Volume 5, Number 2, a publication of Wellness Councils of America (welcoa.org). 2006.

employers with membership in the Wellness Councils of America. There, a trio of fundamental assumptions were replaced with new conventional wisdom.

Old CW (traditional weight-loss paradigm): *Everyone needs to be thin for good health and happiness.* New CW (Health at Every Size): Thin is not intrinsically healthy and beautiful, nor is fat intrinsically unhealthy and unappealing.

Old CW: *People who are not thin are overweight because they have no willpower, eat too much, and don't move enough.* New CW: People naturally have different body shapes and sizes and different preferences for physical activity.

Old CW: *Everyone can be thin, happy and healthy by dieting.* New CW: Dieting usually leads to weight gain, decreased self-esteem and increased risk for disordered eating. Health and happiness grow from the interaction among mental, social, spiritual and physical considerations.[197]

The science behind HAES had been well-established by dozens of rigorous studies and made accessible in important, under-read books by William Bennett and Joel Gurin, Glenn A. Gaesser, Paul Campos, J. Eric Oliver, Linda Bacon, Gina Kolata, Abigail C. Saguy, Carl J. Lavie and Harriet Brown. Please see the footnote and buy several copies for you and your friends of every size, including the thin ones who may think you are fat, dumb and lazy.[198]

Reviewing hundreds of studies, this militia of medical doctors, social scientists and health journalists independently reached the same conclusion: that the causal relationship between increased weight and poor health -- like the contribution of weight loss to improved health — had been largely misrepresented or disproved. And they contend a major and widespread negative consequence has been an unjustified pressure on health professionals

---

197: Jon Robison, PhD, MS. "Health at Every Size: Shifting The Focus To Health." Absolute Advantage, Volume 5, Number 2, a publication of Wellness Councils of America (welcoa.org). 2006.

198: Visit my web site www.fatsmart.org for Amazon links to all of these highly recommended books: William Bennett and Joel Gurin, *The Dieter's Dilemma: Eating Less and Weighing More* (1982). Glenn A. Gaesser, *Big Fat Lies: The Truth About Your Weight and Your Health*, 2002. Paul Campos, *The Obesity Myth: Why America's Obsession with Weight is Hazardous to Your Health*, 2004. J. Eric Oliver, *Fat Politics: The Real Story Behind America's Obesity Epidemic*, 2006. Linda Bacon, *Health At Every Size: The Surprising Truth About Your Weight*, 2010. Gina Kolata, *Rethinking Thin: The New Science of Weight Loss--and the Myths and Realities of Dieting*, 2008. Abigail C. Saguy, *What's Wrong With Fat?* 2013. Carl J. Lavie, *The Obesity Paradox: When Thinner Means Sicker and Heavier Means Healthier*, 2014. Harriet Brown, *Body of Truth: How Science, History, and Culture Drive Our Obsession with Weight -- and What We Can Do About It*, 2016.

to focus on a patient's weight above all else. In order to "First do no harm," HAES-minded healthcare calls on physicians to directly treat specific illnesses while supporting a healthy attitude about weight.

ANY SIZE, FIVE PRINCIPLES

So, who, what, and why is HAES and what are they selling? Is it an all-encompassing brand for miracle fat-blockers, smoothie machines and gym clubs? Big fat no.

In 2003, a California-based steering committee formed a group to be called the Association for Size Diversity and Health. They began with a set of Health At Every Size® principles already making the rounds. Ten years later, as the HAES model was gaining wider acceptance (and a few critics), leadership of the Association for Size Diversity and Health organized a thorough review and revisions to better address political, social and economic changes affecting access to healthcare. Input came from medical professionals, health educators, nutritionists, psychologists, fitness trainers, social workers and more. They worked hard, and it shows.

The Health At Every Size® Principles[199]

1. Weight Inclusivity: Accept and respect the inherent diversity of body shapes and sizes and reject the idealizing or pathologizing of specific weights.

2. Health Enhancement: Support health policies that improve and equalize access to information and services, and personal practices that improve human well-being, including attention to individual physical, economic, social, spiritual, emotional, and other needs.

3. Respectful Care: Acknowledge our biases, and work to end weight discrimination, weight stigma, and weight bias. Provide information and services from an understanding that socio-economic status, race, gender, sexual orientation, age, and other identities impact weight stigma, and support environments that address these inequities.

199: "The Health At Every Size® Approach." Association for Size Diversity and Health. Undated. www. sizediversityandhealth.org. ©2018 ASDAH All Rights Reserved.

4. Eating for Well-being: Promote flexible, individualized eating based on hunger, satiety, nutritional needs, and pleasure, rather than any externally regulated eating plan focused on weight control.

5. Life-Enhancing Movement: Support physical activities that allow people of all sizes, abilities, and interests to engage in enjoyable movement, to the degree that they choose.

Let's double back for a moment to that first rule's direction that no weight should be *pathologized*. That's another way of evoking *medicalization* or, to get down and dirty, *disease mongering*.

Consider shyness, for example. Viewed through the lens of psychology or sociology, being shy is just how some people are in some situations. Somewhere along the continuum between minor shyness and a sweaty, heart-thumping panic attack, a timid human characteristic becomes "social anxiety disorder." And there's a pill for that, possibly prescribed by a physician whose entire staff was recently treated to box lunches by an attractive sales representative for the pharmaceutical company that sells that pill.

Weight, we know, can also reach challenging extremes, from the 68-pound woman with an eating disorder to the 600-pound man who needs piano movers, a crane and a truck to get to a hospital. But the ASDAH sticks to Principle No. 1. "When a weight-specific lens is applied to health, the myriad contributing factors affecting an individual's well-being are usually lost," the group says in its supporting documents. "Improving a person's health is a process that begins by contemplating what it would take to make certain determinants of health available and accessible to different individuals, and not by pathologizing any specific weight."[200]

The Association for Size Diversity and Health also rejects *healthism*, a pejorative used to describe any social or political policy that attempts to impose norms of a so-called healthy lifestyle. "Unfortunately, 'health' is one of a long list of categories that our culture tends to use to value an individual's worth, along with appearance, size, weight, age, ability, gender, race, and others," it says in its statement of purpose. "Healthist judgments have also crept into our

---

200: *The Health At Every Size® Approach.* Association for Size Diversity and Health. Undated. www. sizediversityandhealth.org.

discourse around public health, with spiraling healthcare costs being implicitly or explicitly blamed on the so-called 'choices' of various groups, including fat people."

ASDAH principles reject judgments about individual *responsibility* for health in favor of a focus on individualized health *needs*. This is justifiable, the group argues, because many of the factors that determine our health are not individual in nature. Social, political, and cultural factors -- including poverty, access, and all forms of stigma -- may have an even greater impact on health outcomes than individual choices.

"On a collective level, we support creating health-promoting environments and removing barriers to access. On an individual level, we seek to empower people to engage in those personal practices that best support health and well-being for the individual. There should be no judgment about what people choose to do (or not do) to enhance their well-being," ASDAH believes.[201]

I appreciate that most Americans are fiercely protective of their freedom and proudly embrace the virtues of sacrifice and self-reliance that make every day a Flag Day. But it's also true that the jump in obesity rates exactly dovetails with the rise of the all-American, profit-driven obesogenic environment.

Most businesses have to absorb their real costs of doing business, whether it's taxes, payroll, utilities or waste management. Industries which process and market sugars, salts and fats into low-nutrition trifles are netting billions of dollars. Yet they have been allowed to shrug off their biggest cost of doing business: the bullying, discrimination, self-loathing, and additional health care costs borne by their best customers. They blithely attribute any ill effects of their products to free-willed consumers who *choose* to heed their non-stop urging to eat and drink more.

Public health means everyone's health. Our healthcare system is too big, too complicated, and too expensive to separate the winners and losers with a line on a BMI chart. No one should face an arbitrary weight-based roadblock in pursuit of better health. Instead of extending a leg to trip on, policymakers

---

201: . ASDAH is the authority on *Health At Every Size®*. They deserve credit for hashing out the details of a responsible HAES® approach. Also, it's fun to use the little ® symbol, which helps keep evil corporations from sneaking HAES into their packaging or advertising. Check out their website, and also haescommunity.com.

should offer a helping hand. We've got room for some new values. Health At Every Size seems like a good way to promote liberty and justice for *all*.

SCIENCE. THAT'S WHY.

For those who prefer a good stack of peer-reviewed facts to a warm-and-fuzzy plea for compassion and inclusion, the research just keeps on a-comin'.

Medical care that prioritizes weight loss over attention to genuine health issues is ineffective and often contributes to dangerous weight cycling, eating disorders and heightened weight stigma. So says a massive review of research that was conducted by Ohio State University Psychologist Tracy L. Tylka, together with global associates from California to Great Britain and Iceland.

Drawing on 167 cited studies and reports, they compared traditional "weight-normative" protocols to "weight-inclusive" treatment which prioritize a patient's well-being. Their findings were published in 2014 in the Journal of Obesity:[202]

All health care professionals should play a part in helping patients to overcome body shame and internalized weight stigma, the researchers recommend. And when patients specifically ask for advice to lose weight, a "Do no harm" response should be a holistic approach that gives equal weight to emotional, physical, nutritional, social and spiritual health.

Team Tylka concludes that because weight loss is usually unsustainable and linked to negative consequences, "we argue that it is *unethical* to continue to prescribe weight loss to patients and communities as a pathway to health."[203]

Linda Bacon, Ph.D, a City College of San Francisco professor with advanced degrees in psychotherapy, exercise science, physiology, nutrition and weight regulation, weighed in with her 2008 book with the git-er-done title of "Health At Every Size: The Surprising Truth About Your Weight." In 2014, Bacon followed up with "Body Respect: What Conventional Health Books Get Wrong, Leave Out or Just Plain Fail to Understand About Weight."

202: Tracy L. Tylka and others. "The Weight-Normative versus Weight-Normative Approach to Health: Evaluating the Evidence for Prioritizing Well-Being Over Weight Loss." Journal of Obesity. Volume 2014, Article ID 983495.

203: Tylka and others.

The author brought fresh research to the table. In a study published in the Journal of the American Dietetic Association, Bacon and colleagues enlisted a test group of 78 obese women, all of them wounded veterans of the diet wars. Randomly divided into two groups and assembled for weekly meetings over six months, half of the group received typical diet counseling while the others were instructed in the principle of intuitive eating and health at every size. That was followed by six monthly follow-up sessions.

Do I really need to tell you how this turned out?

Well, for starters, 41 percent of the dieting group dropped out of the study within the first six months, compared to only 8 percent of the HAES group. At the end of the first year, the remaining members of the diet group had indeed lost more weight and showed improvement in several measures of physical and emotional health. After two years, however, the two groups were easily distinguished. Dieters regained weight and retained few health gains. The Health at Every Size group maintained their weight, but sustained improvements in all other measures -- BMI, blood pressure, blood lipids, energy expenditure, eating restraint and self-esteem.[204]

"Quit hassling patients about their weight. Stop prescribing weight loss," Bacon tells the medical community. "Encourage people of all sizes to change focus from weight to health. Support everyone in appreciating their bodies and incorporating healthy lifestyle habits." [205]

UNEASE WITH DISEASE

That new way of thinking about weight almost — *almost* — had a big impact on American medicine in 2013 when delegates to the annual meeting of the American Medical Association took up whether obesity itself is a disease. The matter had been thoroughly studied over the previous year by the AMA's own Council of Science and Public Health, which shared it's detailed reasons both for and against disease status at the Chicago convention. One reason given to declare obesity a disease is that it would reduce the stigma of obesity, muting

204: Linda Bacon, MA, Phd, et al. "Size Acceptance and Intuitive Eating Improve Health for Obese, Female Chronic Dieters." Journal of the American Dietetic Association. Volume 105, Issue 6, Pages 929-936 (June 2005).
205: Bacon, Linda, MA, PhD. "End the War on Obesity: Make Peace With Your Patients." Transcript of a video commentary for Medscape General Medicine. Posted November 27, 2006, http://medgenmed. medscape.com

the perception that heavy people just don't understand the "eat less, move more" solution that supposedly works for everyone.

Ultimately, the study group recommended against the disease classification, primarily because the body mass index routinely used a yardstick for health is so unreliable. They noted, just as you learned in the early pages of this book, that obese patients may exhibit good metabolic indicators, just as normal weight people may test poorly for the same benchmarks. Opponents also argued that medicalizing obesity would define a third of Americans as being ill and encourage more reliance on surgery or costly drugs.

But AMA members at large were more persuaded by groups favoring the classification, including associations representing cardiologists and endocrinologists. And so they adopted a resolution declaring obesity as a "metabolic and hormonal disease state" that leads to Type 2 diabetes and cardiovascular disease.[206]

An association's resolution is not civil law, of course, but the AMA's vote is expected to have implications for international medicine, U.S. public policy, and — nitty-grittiest of all — how willing public and private insurers are to pay for treatments. The Affordable Care Act of 2010 already included provisions for certain obesity prevention and treatment programs, but only eight states were fully on board with related Medicaid coverage, according to one study.

The push to medicalize obesity may help standardize treatments and reimbursements, something the billion-dollar bean-counters of the healthcare and weight-loss industries are looking forward to. "In other words, follow the money," writes Harriet Brown. If Medicare fully implements coverage of obesity as a disease, she says, "doctors who even mention weight to their patients could charge more for the same visit than doctors who don't."[207]

EXPRESS YOURSELF

At a minimum, it's good the medical establishment had an open debate about putting the disease label on obesity. I like to think most health providers

---

206: Andrew Pollack. "A.M.A. Recognizes Obesity as a Disease." Nytimes.com. June 18, 2013.

207: Harriet Brown. "How Obesity Became A Disease." Theatlantic.com. March 24, 2015. Adapted from Brown's 2016 book, "Body of Truth: How Science, History, and Culture Drive Our Obsession With Weight – And What We Can Do About It."

will honor any patient's sincere preference for a holistic evaluation and treatment of their health needs. But as medical practices, large and small, are being pushed to accept the BMI-based medicalization of weight, patients must be prepared to clearly express that desire and be prepared to switch to a more-receptive practitioner.

To adopt and advocate for HAES principles means firmly confronting deeply held personal beliefs and institutionalized opposition. Not sure you can find the right words? Among the many resources in Bacon's *Health At Every Size* book are some sample letters to help express your HAES philosophy.[208]

"Trumpeting obesity concerns and admonishing people to lose weight is not just misguided, but downright damaging," Bacon writes in a sample letter to health care providers.

By adapting Bacon's templates, you'll be convincingly prepared to also make your case to friends and family, work associates caught in the diet yo-yo cycle, school administrators and teachers, elected officials and special interest groups. Before long, you may be running for Congress or grabbing the mic from the U.S. Surgeon General. But start small and consider all the changes you'd have to personally accept to become a single HAES success story. Start with a check-up and chat with your physician about the principles of Health at Every Size. Get some baseline measurements of your health to compare after a year, two years and forever. Connect with laymen and professionals on social media. Start a HAES support and advocacy group. Take advantage of a formal curriculum based on the principles.[209] Shout to be heard over the powerful presence of the diet and fitness industry.

Enjoy food. Enjoy movement. Live your dreams. Take the DVR of your life off *pause* and move forward at X2 speed.

In the months to come, you can get positive reinforcement and enabling information from all the good books I've mentioned here. While I am a mere

---

208: Linda Bacon, PhD. Health at Every Size: The Surprising Truth About Your Weight. BenBella Books, Inc. Dallas, TX. 2008, with additional material from the author in 2010.
209: The Association for Size Diversity and Health (ASDAH), the National Association to Advance Fat Acceptance (NAAFA), and the Society for Nutrition Education and Behavior (SNEB) offer a Health At Every Size® Curriculum for the education of college and university students and health profession-als. For more information on the program and its sponsors, make the internet rounds at haescommunity.com, haescurriculum.com and sizediversityandhealth.org.

journalist with an overdose of opinions, they are the experts upon whose shoulders I wobbly stand.

And what a bonus! The cherry on a sundae will come when tens, hundreds — millions? -- of Americans choose to focus on health and self-acceptance as the path to coming out of the closet as proudly *Fat, Smart and Happy*.

17

WHAT TO EAT!

What to eat? What, with regard to health and longevity, to eat? What exactly?

The best choice, although not always the most obvious choice, is food. Real food. Something your great-grandmother would have eaten. Or a brawny rail splitter. Or your grandmother, especially if she was a brawny rail splitter.

Proving he was neither politician nor bureaucrat, popular writer-omnivore Michael Pollan famously reduced all the best nutrition advice to just seven words: "Eat food, not too much, mostly plants."

By food, he means real food, not the processed, re-imagined Frankenfoods that have seized entire aisles of food stores everywhere. Leave that stuff for the walking dead. They'll eat anything, even well beyond expiration dates.

The great joy and convenience of eating healthy whole foods is that serving sizes and satiety both come naturally, no measurements or calculations required. Balance is still important, but every meal doesn't have to represent all food groups. Keep it close to balanced over a period of a few days and your body will think you're a genius. If you go overboard on empty calories one day, jump into a burning lake of fire the next day as an inspiring act of penance. Or just make some offsetting adjustments in caloric intake. Don't act like a bloodied martyr when the time is right to decline a warm croissant or bagel with cream cheese. There will be many croissant and bagel days still to come.

Eat a good breakfast, lunch and dinner, and plan a healthy snack before it's an emergency. Eat slowly. Enjoy what's on your plate before it's in your mouth. Eat and move to be healthier at your present weight. And if you happen to slowly lose weight . . . you get to buy some new clothes.

Are you afraid to taste healthy foods?. When you find yourself thinking "Yuck, not that, not me," remember this: We were all born with a preference for mother's milk alone. But we grow up and we learn to like new foods. We add heat, salt and pepper and the bitter white onion becomes caramelized, sweet, golden and delicious.

Still, I wonder why and when the first brave soul tried eating a gnarly green and purple sprout of asparagus, some squishy squid, ominous oysters, the tongue of a cow or the unraveled and rinsed intestines of a hog.

I'm content knowing none of us has to personally find out if potential edibles are deadly. Today, being bold, *Fat, Smart and Happy* simply means going where millions of people have gone before you, and I don't mean Pizza Hut. Practically everything a healthy body needs is available year-round, fresh or frozen, along the perimeter walls of your neighborhood grocery store.

Except where noted, most of the following information is drawn from the USDA's 2015 Dietary Guidelines[210] and the less politicized Harvard T.H. Chan School of Public Health's excellent website.[211] Take those two sources, add a pinch of common sense, and you've got the foundation of a solid grocery shopping list for this week and forever.

PROTEIN

We are roundly aware of how effortlessly our bodies are able to store fats and carbohydrates for that possible future famine. Not so with protein, or, more accurately, the 20 or so amino acids which are genetically directed to make up the proteins we carry around as tissue, bones, and muscle. Nutritionists say we need to freshly ingest healthy proteins every day. As to how much, there is less agreement, but 50 to 100 grams a day is in the easy-to-score ballpark. Converted to ounces, that's . . . well, too complicated.

210: *https://health.gov/dietaryguidelines/2015/*
211: *https://www.hsph.harvard.edu/nutritionsource.*

Just think of it this way: Adults need about six ounces of protein a day. Each of the following counts as one-ounce serving of protein: a cup of milk, one egg or two egg whites, a tablespoon of peanut butter, a fourth-cup of dried beans, a half-ounce of nuts or seeds, or an ounce of cooked fish, poultry or beef.

Skimping on protein is just one of many bad ideas associated with trying to lose weight quickly. Getting enough protein is easy. The trick is to not rely on fatty or processed meats. A broiled 6-ounce porterhouse steak provides 38 grams of complete protein -- along with 44 grams of fat, 16 of them saturated. Lordy, that's lardy. Compare that to a cup of 1% low-fat milk, which provides 8 grams of protein with only 2.5 grams of fat.

An 8-ounce sirloin a day will not keep the doctor away. Daily consumption of red meat is strongly associated with increased risk of cardiovascular disease, diabetes, and cancer. So make peace with all the other protein options, especially beans and peas, which do double duty as vegetables.

Satisfying sources of protein abound. Three ounces of canned tuna provide 20 grams; a roasted, skinless chicken breast has 26 grams. Other fish and shellfish are also delicious packages for protein.

Vegans need not go hungry. Dried beans and peas, nuts and seeds deliver protein directly from the earth to you. Black beans, lentils, almonds, cashews and hazelnuts are all good amino acid sources, a/k/a the building blocks of protein.

Nevertheless, animal sources have the most complete protein, while other food sources tend to lack one or more of the "essential" amino acids. The simple and satisfying work-around is to enjoy a wide variety of protein-rich foods. That is doubly true for vegetarians.

In the late 1990s, soybeans and soy-based foods took on some marketing magic when preliminary studies suggested soy protein could help reduce cholesterol, prevent breast and prostate cancer, aid weight loss, and chill hot flashes. But Harvard's nutritionists now say many of those claims have been tempered by further study. They put soybeans and tofu in the "eat in moderation" category, suggesting just two to four servings a week, while avoiding supplements with concentrated soy protein altogether. Heavily processed or fermented soy products have also been linked to migraine headaches.

Carnivores can minimize guilt and maximize the health benefits of meats by choosing leaner cuts of meats, and keeping them lean in the preparation process. A marbled, buttered and fried steak doesn't fit the bill. Avoid the heavily processed, high-fat luncheon meats altogether. They're normally packed with extra salt and preservatives, so good riddance. Choose lean cuts of beef, whether sliced or ground. Chicken and turkey are nutritious and versatile choices, but remove the skin before cooking. Spices and a little olive oil will provide ample flavor.

Speaking of frying: don't. Any lean cut of meat will be delicious when seasoned, then broiled, grilled or poached. Use a spoon or paper towel to soak up any rendered fat.

Remember that protein is a weight watcher's best friend because it satisfies hunger longer than any other food group. It's just the opposite of a sugar high and crash. In one University of Washington study, a group of slightly overweight people were put on a diet low in fat with about double the typical amount of calories coming from protein. Participants, while losing weight, voiced a common complaint. They felt *too full*.

Other studies have produced similar findings. Protein satisfies. And satiety is your body trying to tell you, "You've had enough to eat. Now brush your teeth and walk the dog."

DAIRY

"Milk: Two Glasses A Day Tones Muscles, Keeps the Fat Away in Women, Study Shows."[212]

That was the headline for a news release published on a fairly respected website featuring "the latest research news." But when I printed it out for future reference I penciled in some dollar signs to remind me of the source. The 2010 $tudy looked at a small group of women who drank two glasses of milk instead of a sugary energy drink -- *after their weight-lifting routine*. It was financed in part by Dairy Farmers of Canada.

212: "Milk: Two Glasses A Day Tones Muscles, Keeps the Fat Away In Women, Study Shows." *Science Daily.com.* May 28, 2010.

God bless those dairy farmers. They put in a half-day of work before I even roll out of bed. But, as I have emphasized repeatedly, when money talks, veracity walks, and that includes any "independent" study financed even partially by a for-profit company or trade organization.

You can't blame Canadian dairymen for making the effort. Their U.S. counterparts have been getting great mileage for years from advertising campaigns powered by inconclusive or ethically tainted studies. The (U.S.) National Dairy Council spent about $200 million on a "3-A-Day" promotion suggesting a connection between regular milk drinking and weight loss.

But a 2005 investigation by Associated Press writer J.M. Hirsch found the industry claims were based largely on research it had helped finance. The studies centered around research by Michael Zemel, a University of Tennessee nutritionist who had received more than $2 million in research funding from the Dairy Council.[213]

Independent experts told Hirsch that Zemel's basic research was solid, but the industry's advertised conclusions leapfrogged the available data. Even Zemel agreed his work was often misunderstood. It's not as simple as (1.) drink milk, (2.) lose weight, he told the AP. Instead, Zemel said the prescription only works for people who eat a low-calorie diet and who are not already having three servings a day of dairy.[214]

A more recent study may have come closer to identifying the real merits of consuming dairy products, although the results were misconstrued by many media outlets as a straight-up connection between drinking milk and weight loss. The research conducted at Israel's Ben-Gurion University and published in 2010 in the American Journal of Clinical Nutrition "proved," according to press releases, "that people on a diet who consumed more milk or dairy products lost more weight on average than those who consumed little or no milk." [215, 216]

In fact, the study was financed in part by a private foundation and only suggested the intake of calcium and vitamin D *associated* with dairy consumption

213: J.M. Hirsch, Associated Press. "Link Between Dairy, Weight Loss Unclear." *USA Today.* July 17, 2005.
214: Hirsch.
215: "Lose Weight By Drinking Milk." *news.softpedia.com.* September 21, 2010.
216: Danit R. Shahar and others. "Dairy Calcium Intake, Serum Vitamin D, and Successful Weight Loss." *American Journal of Clinical Nutrition.* September 1, 2010.

may contribute to weight loss. Britain's National Health Service found several shortcomings in the research and concluded "there is not sufficient evidence from this study to suggest dairy has a direct effect on weight loss."[217]

Dairy may be optional, but calcium and Vitamin D are two gotta-haves. When the dairy industry tells you calcium is important for bone health, they've slipped a whole truth into the usual glass of skimmed facts. Many Americans have low bone mass, putting them at risk of osteoporosis and bone fractures. Adolescent girls, adult women and 50-something adults are most likely to need more calcium. And everyone needs the stuff to maintain the health of muscles, blood vessels, and nerves.

We know vitamin D is important to health because we have names for conditions related to deficiencies. In adults, the softening of bones is called osteomalacia. Among children, the condition is called rickets. (It's the same thing, but more fun to say aloud. "Want to play football?" "Naw, I can't today. Got rickets." And what if the Health Police wrote up citations for vitamin D deficiency? Why, we'd soon have street protesters organizing to picket rickets tickets.)

Vitamin D plays several roles in promoting health. Because it promotes calcium absorption, it's no surprise that vitamin D and calcium are added together to many processed foods. As for weight loss, a very small study at the University of Minnesota suggested that calorie-cutting was less effective among those with insufficient vitamin D levels.

So, if calcium and vitamin D are both important to health and weight management, but dairy products contain excessive amounts of fat, then the smart thing to do is . . . drink more whole milk and eat more cheese? Yes and yes, according to a Swedish study and the USDA.

After tracking the eating habits of 19,352 women for nine years, researchers at Stockholm's Karolinska Institute determined, among other things, that women who had regularly consumed full-fat milk or cheese had a lower BMI than the rest of the group. Based on their findings, researchers said their "surprising conclusion" was that a glass of whole milk every day will result in 15

217: "Behind the Headlines: Dairy Diet." United Kingdom National Health Service. *nhs.uk.news* September 17, 2010.

percent less weight gain. Full-fat cheese was twice as effective, with a portion a day associated with a 30 percent less weight gain.[218] The study, published in the *American Journal of Clinical Nutrition,* considered several explanations for the inverse correlation between dairy fat consumption and weight loss, but reached few conclusions other than to *rule out* calcium intake as a significant factor in weight loss. [219]

Given all the confusion and conflicting studies about the relative benefits of dairy foods and milk fat, it's a given that different agencies within the U.S. Department of Agriculture would take bipolar positions on such weighty, political matters.

For years, the nutrition-focused side of the USDA has urged Americans to reduce their consumption of saturated fats and therefore to choose no-fat or low-fat versions of milk and cheese. That effort has had a major impact on milk-buying habits.

At the same time, Dairy Management, a marketing arm of the USDA underwritten by dairymen, has been equally influential, working directly with restaurant chains such as Domino's Pizza and Taco Bell to introduce more menu items with more and more cheese.[220]

In one year, Dairy Management spent $136 Million -- about 20 times the budget for USDA's healthy diet promotion arm. When the New York Times reported on the internal conflict, the USDA's response was a big, fat "No comment."[221]

Maybe these stats say it all: Americans now consume, on average, 36 pounds of cheese a year, nearly three times the rate in 1970. Cheese now represents almost half of all dairy products consumed in the U.S. And cheese is the largest source of saturated fat (about 30 percent) in the American diet. And it's delicious.

218: "Full Fat Milk Makes You Thinner -- Swedish Study." *www.thelocal.se* (The Local: Sweden's News in English) *January 8, 2007.*
219: Rosell, Magdalena, Niclas N. Hakansson, and Alicja Wolk. "Association Between Dairy Food Consumption and Weight Change Over 9 y in 19,352 Perimenopausal Women." *The American Journal of Clinical Nutrition.* 2006.
220: Michael Moss. "While Warning About Fat, U.S. Pushes Cheese Sales." *The New York Times.* November 6, 2010.
221: Moss.

Do we need dairy products at all? For a great many adults who are lactose intolerant, the body's answer is an invisible, generously scented flatulence. Nutritionist Marion Nestle points out that in many parts of the world where cow's milk is not a regular part of the diet, people have fewer bone problems than we do, and they maintain a good calcium balance on less than half the calcium intake we're advised to consume. Calcium retention, she says, is influenced by the overall diet -- too much protein and salt, not enough plant sources -- as well as levels of exercise, alcohol, and smoking.[222]

And then there are the ethical issues that accompany the heavily industrialized production of milk today. The dairy business is one that depends on genetic manipulation, powerful hormones and four or five years of regular cow insemination to induce continuous pregnancy. Weaned calves can look forward to crowded feedlots, intensive milking, and painful mastitis. Got Milk? Check. Got Guilt? I do now.

To get you to drink industrial milk, food scientists step in to complicate what should be a simple, whole food. To maintain a creamy texture in low-fat milk, commercial dairies resort to additives, including powdered milk rich in unhealthy oxidized cholesterol. That's the upside. The takeaway is the reduction of the milk fat the body needs to absorb fat-soluble vitamins.

The USDA's 2015 Dietary Guidelines still recommend regular consumption of fat-free and low-fat dairy products, including milk, yogurt and cheese. Children should have the equivalent of two cups a day. Age nine and up can have three cups a day, the feds say. Harvard's School of Public Health agrees that calcium intake is important, but cautions against milk because of its saturated fats. It suggests non-dairy sources of calcium, including collards, bok choy, fortified soy milk or supplements with both calcium and vitamin D.

I am sorry to have given you so much contradictory information about the merits of milk. This one's a real head-scratcher. But here's what I think: If you like milk -- and it likes you -- then don't be afraid to enjoy the occasional glass of whole milk, preferably from a reputable, ethical and organic processor. Regardless, a good balance of whole foods will fill in most nutrition gaps.

222: Marion. Nestle. *What to Eat*. New York: *North Point Press*. 2006., p. 74.

WHOLE GRAINS AND FIBER

American farmland was planted in 2016 with 143 million acres of nourishing whole-grain corn and wheat. When it arrived in our restaurants and grocery aisles, most of it had been murdered and mutilated, then caked in cosmetics to conceal the carnage.

Oh, it keeps us fueled and running, but with all the knocks and pings of watered-down gasoline. Among 97 food categories defined in the Dietary Guidelines for Americans, most of our top 10 sources of calories were grain-based, including desserts (cakes, cookies, donuts, granola bars), yeast breads, soft drinks and sports drinks, alcoholic beverages, pizza, pasta, tortillas and tacos. Instead of grainy goodness, these staples of the American diet are often stripped of nutrients, then flavored with fats and sugars.

Whole grains include the entire grain seed, or kernel, which comprises the bran, germ, and endosperm. The names alone can be unappetizing, but whole grains are a steady source of nutrients such as iron, magnesium, selenium, B vitamins and varying amounts of dietary fiber. There's also evidence that whole grains are associated with lower body weight and reduced risk of heart disease and diabetes. So whole grain is a good thing, and not just limited to corn and wheat. Rolled oats, brown or wild race, barley, and rye all start life as nutritious whole grains.

But food processors, in their never-ending quest to make all human chow palatable to four-year-olds, employ an arsenal of chemical and mechanical techniques to turn good grain over to The Dark Side. After milling grain to remove the germ and bran, the so-called refined grain has a finer texture and longer shelf life, while sacrificing important dietary fiber, iron and B vitamins. Then refiners re-add some vitamins and minerals, and call it enriched grain.

The 2010 and 2015 health.gov Dietary Guidelines provide advice that is easier to understand than it is to follow: At least half of all grains consumed should be whole grains. Increase whole grain intake by replacing refined grains with whole grains. You will find that most of the breads in the grocery touting whole wheat on the front of the package also have a long list of processed grains in the ingredients panel.

Americans certainly don't have any trouble including refined or enriched grains in their diets, consuming on average more than twice the recommended three ounces a day. Mostly, it comes from breads, pizza, grain-based desserts, tortillas, burritos, tacos and pasta.

Another penalty for trying to fill up with junk grains is that most Americans get barely half the recommended 20–35 grams of dietary fiber per day. That's just dumb, because dietary fiber contributes greatly to a feeling of fullness and the body's ability to absorb nutrients, both of which help promote a healthy body weight.

You may have to visit a hipster bakery to find genuine whole wheat bread. Stock up, freeze a few bags, and you'll have it when you need it. My breakfast is often one hearty slice, toasted, with butter and honey or molasses, or peanut butter, or cream cheese with nuts and berries. Delish, and I'm not sleepy afterwards or in a hurry for lunch.

The federal MyPlate graphic wisely recommends that three-fourths of your plate should have fiber-rich grains, fruits and vegetables. And you know that doesn't mean heavily processed, sweetened or fried. It means real food with real flavor and nutrients. Remember, frozen fruits and vegetables are super okay to use year-round. They are nearly identical in nutrients to their fresh counterparts along the produce aisle. Yet they are usually less expensive than their fresh peers, in-season year-round, and shielded from the indignation of other shoppers' sneezing and squeezing.

SALT AND SODIUM

"Americans spend more than $15 billion each year on drugs to treat hypertension, yet the government spends almost nothing to reduce salt consumption." [223]

That appeal to inject common sense and kitchen table economics into national policy was made more than a decade ago by Michael F. Jacobson, co-founder and president of the nonprofit Center for Science in the Public Interest. Echoing numbers issued by the U.S. Center for Disease Control, the consumer

---

223: ""Forgotten Killer" Salt Kills 150,000 a Year, Says CSPI Report." February 24, 2005 prepared statement from the Center for Science in the Public Interest.

group said too much salt in the diet is boosting Americans' blood pressure and is "prematurely killing" tens of thousands of us.

To add action to words, the CSPI filed a federal suit aimed at compelling the Food and Drug Administration to classify salt as a food additive. That means salt would no longer rest in the comfortable, loosely regulated FDA food category of "Generally Recognized as Safe."

This portrait of salt as a food villain is certainly a late-blooming concept for humanity. Historically, trade routes and fortunes were built on moving tons of the stuff around the world.

"But I hardly use any salt at all," you're thinking. "I don't even clean out the shaker top when half of the holes are clogged. And I add a lot of different spices in the kitchen, but just a pinch of salt."

Well, good for you! You're probably not getting too much salt in your diet, unless perhaps you also enjoy soy sauce, mustard, ketchup and salad dressings, or your day wouldn't be complete without some potato chips, tomato juice, salsa, pretzels, bread, pasta, pizza, chicken, cold cuts, cheese, sausage, tacos, beef, pork or a big ol' dill pickle!

The 2015 Dietary Guidelines for most Americans are unchanged from 2005 and 2010 versions. They recommend limiting daily sodium intake to less than 2,300 milligrams. But for half of the American population, the recommendation is a daily limit of 1,500 mg. That now applies to children, as well as adults over age 51 in general, and specifically to all African-Americans and those people with high blood pressure, diabetes or chronic kidney disease.

The problem, as the CSPI and most public health advocates agree, is that most Americans consume between 3,500 and 4,000 mg of sodium per day, or twice the recommended amounts.

True, one could add a single teaspoon of table salt to foods prepared at home and rack up 2,300 mg of sodium. But Joe and Jane Typical only get about 5 percent of their daily sodium intake from salt added during cooking, and another 6 percent sprinkled at the table. All the rest -- and that's a lot -- comes from the packaged and processed foods found on every aisle of the food market, and from restaurants, where a penny's worth of salt is a time-honored way to kick up flavors and make you thirsty for a second beer or endless refills of sugary drinks.

Leave it to the nutritionists at heath.gov to create a pie made entirely from salt. In this case the pie is included in the 2015 dietary guidelines for Americans. It slices up our typical sodium intake by food source and looks like this:

Most away-from-home food comes with a free side order of sodium. McDonald's has 10 or more sandwiches with at least 1,500 mg of sodium -- 11 counting the breakfast bagel with steak, egg and cheese. Taco Bell's Smothered Beef Burrito comes with 2,260 mg of sodium; Sonic's large Chili Cheese Tots tops that with 2,760 mg; Hardee's 2/3 pound Monster Thickburger comes with a lot of everything, including 95 grams of fat and 2,820 mg of sodium. For a while, at least, Pizza Hut topped one 2016 search for the saltiest food by offering a 9-inch Meat Lovers PANormous "personal" Pizza capable of transmitting 3,670 mg of sodium.[224]

Popular restaurants with real plates and waiters rarely skimp on the salt. Olive Garden's lunch and dinner menu includes 38 items with 1,500 mg or more. Take their Tour of Italy entree (3,250 mg) with a House Salad with dressing (740 mg) and two garlic-butter bread sticks (460 mg each) and you've got a meal with 4,910 mg of sodium.

Applebee's long and tempting menu is one more salt flat along your favorite retail highway. The menu has 74 opportunities to score 1,500-plus milligrams of sodium, including 18 appetizers, two of which have more than 6,000 mg each. All six of Applebee's featured light meals under 640 calories contain a full day's worth of sodium, as do all six of their featured salads with dressing. Other standouts in and around shopping malls include Chili's Boneless Buffalo Chicken Salad, 3,730 mg of sodium; Cheesecake Factory's Sunrise Fiesta Burrito, 4,600 mg; and, perhaps the saltiest dish documented in the last few years, PF Chang's Hot & Sour Soup Bowl, with 7,980 mg of sodium.[225] Denny's coffee is still a big draw. Use your own judgment about the 50 or more menu items with at least 1,500 mg of sodium. [226]

224: Dan Myers. The Daily Meal. "America's Saltiest Fast Foods." *Foxnews.com*. February 18, 2016.
225: "The 10 Saltiest Foods in America." By the staff of Eat This, Not That! *(www.eatthis.com)* as re-posted by www.yahoo.com, October 24, 2014.
226: "Activist Group Sues Denny's Over Sodium Levels." July 23, 2009, *Reuters.com*.

All fast food and casual dining chains offer ample opportunities to stitch together a healthy meal, especially for those willing to study the online nutrition information before piling into the SUV. Or anyone can cut the sodium and carbs for any purchased meal by half just by sharing an oversized serving with a friend or take-home box.

Low-salt, like low-fat and low-cal, has joined the ranks of food trends worthy of exploitation. Over the past several years, it's been easier to find items throughout the grocery that have been reformulated with lower sodium. Some were desalted quietly so as not to scare off customers. Campbell's Soup learned that lesson the hard way.

It announced the brand was reducing sodium in one of its soup lines by nearly half. A few years later, "in response to customer feedback" (Translation: a drop in sales), Campbell's announced it would "improve the taste" of about 30 of its canned soups by increasing sodium levels.

Today, most Campbell's soups are still mmm-mmm-salty. Of 296 varieties of soups and broth produced, 52 products (17 percent) meet the FDA heart-healthy recommendation of 480 mg or less of sodium. But that's up from less than 1 percent just a few years earlier. It's a very positive trend, so maybe the less said about it, the better.[227]

THE ALT SALT DEBATE

But what if the Conventional Wisdom about encouraging a reduction in salt intake is like a lot of CW -- essentially flawed? There have been, in fact, several serious studies challenging the magic of the mantra.

A 2010 study by Harvard researchers showed that sodium intake for Americans has remained virtually unchanged for 40 years, even though the population's rate of hypertension has increased substantially. A much broader study covering 19,000-plus subjects in 33 countries over 26 years found a surprising narrow range of sodium intake worldwide and raises the possibility that reducing salt in prepared foods might have the unintended consequence of encouraging higher calorie consumption in an effort to maintain a natural, healthy sodium intake. That's according to some medical researchers with

227: www.campbellnutrition.com

friendly connections to a trade association known as The Salt Institute. Tainted? Probably, but let's recognize also that many of the studies reinforcing the link between sodium and high blood pressure are sponsored by donation-dependent groups that need a recognizable villain.

One pertinent fact often missing from public health debates is that a majority of people are not strongly affected by dietary sodium levels.

At least a fourth of the U.S. population, however, is considered *salt sensitive*. *We're* not talking about how your taste buds react, although there might be a correlation. There's no easy test for salt sensitivity. Age, fitness levels and weight may be factors. The reason all African Americans are cautioned about sodium intake is that nearly three-fourths of blacks are believed to be salt sensitive.

Time out. We can't cherry-pick our nutrients. We eat foods. Yes, sodium levels may be important in controlling high blood pressure, but perhaps not nearly so significant as its interaction with other nutrients, including calcium, magnesium and potassium. As with so much that shapes health and happiness, balance is everything. Scientists haven't nailed down all the specific benefits of magnesium or potassium (and never will as long as there is new grant money to go after), but suspect it helps reduce blood pressure by relaxing tiny blood vessels and/or helping the body flush out excess fluid and sodium.

When it comes to reducing the risk of heart disease, potassium may be the anti-salt. The importance of balance was suggested by a 15-year study of 12,267 U.S. adults. Subjects with the highest ratio of sodium to potassium intake had a 50 percent increased risk of death from any cause and about *twice the risk* of death from heart disease, according to the research team at the U.S. Centers for Disease Control. [228]

Getting the recommended 4,700 milligrams of potassium a day is tasty, affordable and doable. Although bananas get most of the potassium P.R., that 420 mg per servings is less than is provided by a cup of tomato juice (527 mg), a half cup of canned white beans (595 mg), carrot juice (689 mg) or a baked potato with skin (941 mg).

228: Kathleen Doheny. "High-Sodium, Low-Potassium Diet Linked to Heart Risk." *WebMD.com*. July 11, 2011.

All these foods are staples of the basic recommendations in the Dietary Guidelines. For a more directed approach to controlling high blood pressure, just dash on over your local library or internet search box and get familiar with "Dietary Approaches to Stop Hypertension." The so-called DASH diet was developed in the 1990s after clinical trials of three different diets by the National Institute of Health. It's been proven effective at reducing blood pressure, and is now endorsed by the USDA as a smart, well-balanced approach to eating for just about everybody.

Physical activity decreases salt's negative effect on blood pressure. So there you go -- one more reason to get moving. Drinking plenty of water also helps regulate retention of sodium and a million other micro-miracles in the body.

FRUITS AND VEGETABLES

C'mon. You know how important real garden foods are to health and fitness. Fresh is usually best, frozen is nearly identical in nutrition profiles, and canned versions are worthy options if you pay attention to added salts and sugars. See a comprehensive list in the next chapter.

FOODS IN THE NEWS

Several studies have suggested that a daily glass of red wine does a body good. Perhaps it even helps explains the so-called French paradox, the puzzling habit of the French to regularly enjoy high-fat foods with apparent impunity. A titillating 2006 study at Harvard found an unexpected benefit when a group of mice volunteered to ingest a high-fat diet. Interestingly, some of the mice wore little berets and drank little mouse-size glasses of red wine served with tiny wedges of cheese. It was a very cute experiment, so much so that the researchers had to make it sound more science-y to get it published in an academic journal. Instead, they claimed the wine-loving mice were only given a large daily supplement of resveratrol, a natural substance found is in the skin of grapes and in red wine. Sure enough, all the mice on a high-fat diet got fat, but the ones on resveratrol did not have the same enlarged livers or signs of impending diabetes. The mouse gluttons with the grape ingredient also lived longer.

Be advised the amount of resveratrol given the mice was about 300 times what is available in a glass of wine. Still, the research may lead to creation of a useful dietary supplement.

Or maybe the red stuff isn't really what's important. The resident experts at the Harvard School of Public Health have counted more than 100 studies showing an association between moderate drinking, be it beer, wine or booze, and a 25 to 40 percent reduction in risk for heart attack, strokes and other cardiovascular disease. The accepted explanation is that the simple molecules of ethanol found in adult beverages raises the body's levels of HDL cholesterol, the lipoprotein famously associated with improved protection against heart disease.

Too good to be true? Yes, there are caveats aplenty.

"It's safe to say that alcohol is both a tonic and a poison. The difference lies mostly in the dose," Harvard's researchers said in their public statement on the risks and benefits of alcohol.[229]

Gender and genetics are also factors. Women who have two or more drinks a day have about a 40 percent higher rate of developing breast cancer. And men who have three or more drinks in mixed company are more likely to act stupid around women with cleavage. For purposes of this very purposeful book, we should also be interested in the science of beer bellies. Aside from aesthetics, we care because big bellies are an obvious sign of "central adiposity," which is a predictor of cardiovascular disease.

Beer may get more credit for bellies than it deserves. A 2003 study of more than 2,300 men and women showed wine drinking was associated with the least abdominal fat, liquor with the most, and beer with no strong correlation. What matters most, the belly study found, is the when and how much of alcohol consumption. Small amounts of alcohol consumed on a regular basis were associated with the smallest abdomens -- even trimmer than the men and women who didn't drink at all. The guttiest members of the study group were those weekend warriors who only drank occasionally, but in large amounts.[230]

Only a small portion of consumed alcohol is stored as fat. The problem for weight watchers is that most of the alcohol is converted to acetate. Once in the bloodstream, the chemical temporarily trashes the body's normal fat-burning ability. And fat not burned is fat that shows up in the mirror.

229: "Alcohol: Balancing Risks and Benefits." *Harvard School of Public Health.* www.hsph.harvard.edu/ nutritionsource 2007
230: J.M. Dorn and others. "Alcohol Drinking Patterns Differentially Affect Central Adiposity as Measured by Abdomical Height in Women and Men." *Journal of Nutrition.* August 2003.

TEA

Hundreds of studies have been done on the possible health effects of drinking tea. The results, especially for green tea, are largely positive. Brain, heart, and cell health may benefit. Green tea may improve metabolism enough to help keep weight off once you've lost it. Blood sugar levels and blood pressure also may improve. Although tea drinking has been associated with health benefits for centuries, only in recent years have its medicinal properties been investigated scientifically. Tea's good reputation is largely due to its high content of flavonoids — plant-derived compounds that are antioxidants. Studies have found an association between consuming green tea and a reduced risk for several cancers, including, skin, breast, lung, colon, esophageal, and bladder, according to reporting for Harvard Women's Health Watch. Additional benefits for regular consumers of green and black teas include a reduced risk for heart disease. That's because the antioxidants in green, black, and oolong teas can help block the oxidation of bad cholesterol, increase good cholesterol and improve artery function. A Chinese study published in the Archives of Internal Medicine showed a 46 to 65 percent reduction in hypertension risk in regular consumers of oolong or green tea, compared to non-consumers of tea.[231]

Drinking a cup of tea a few times a day helps to absorb its antioxidants and other healthful plant compounds. The best way to get the benefits of tea is to drink it freshly brewed. Allow tea to steep in hot (not boiling) water for three to five minutes to bring out its catechins. Adding a little lemon juice makes tea's healthy compounds easier to absorb; a little milk or cream has the opposite effect. Typical of most processed foods, the decaffeinated, instant or bottled teas have less of the good stuff, including flavor.

COFFEE

If coffee gives you jitters, headaches, brown teeth or frequent trips to the bathroom: Bummer. But if coffee completes you, enjoy it in good health and a clear conscience -- so long as there is more coffee than cream in the cup.

About half the U.S. population drinks coffee every day, making it a significant source of antioxidants. Yes, the aromatic bean renders a cup of

---

231: "Benefit of Drinking Green Tea: The Proof Is In -- Drinking Tea Is Healthy, Says Harvard Women's Health Watch." *Harvard Medical School* press release. September 2004

soothing alertness packed with a shot of antioxidants, much like a normal serving of blueberries, raspberries or grape juice. In the last few years, other studies have shown regular coffee drinking may reduce the risk of heart disease, diabetes, cirrhosis of the liver and certain cancers. It sounds like coffee is achieving more than some people who drink it.

"There's no compelling evidence that shows it's harmful," said one university pharmacologist, "and every day there's more evidence that shows coffee is beneficial."[232]

Decaffeinated coffee has many of the same benefits of the real stuff, including reducing the risk for diabetes. And it won't keep you up late at night. Besides, that's what this book is for.

ANTIOXIDANTS: RIPE OR HYPE?

I've been rather cavalier in dropping the A-word into prior discussions of the health benefits of tea and coffee. Increasingly in paid advertising and on food labels, we are pelted with impassioned reminders to stoke up on antioxidants. But what are they? Are they the real deal?

Let's begin with free radicals. I say put those troublemakers back in jail where they belong!

Let's start over with free radicals. That is also the name scientists give to a variety of naturally occurring chemicals in the body which share a common nasty habit of hijacking electrons from other molecules. Such electron theft can damage cell membranes, insert a "404 Not Found" error message into a strand of DNA, or do something as specific as encouraging bad cholesterol to clog an artery. Antioxidants, then, are the pacifist good guys in the body's battleground, generously giving up their own electrons to thankless free radicals, without damaging themselves. You've heard of many of the chemicals with antioxidant properties: vitamin C, vitamin E, beta-carotene, selenium, manganese, coenzyme Q10, phenols, polyphenols and the one I keep expecting to be co-opted as the brand name for a candy -- flavonoids. Scrupulous readers will correctly recognize this whole atom-splitting analysis reeks of nutritionism.

232: Peter Martin, M.D., director of the Division of Addiction Psychiatry at Vanderbilt University, as quoted by Susan Yara. "Coffee Perks." *Forbes.com.* October 14, 2005.

It did, in fact, take root in the 1990s when researchers began to connect the damage caused by free radicals to heart disease and cancer. Studies had already shown that people who ate plenty of fruits and vegetables were at lower risk for disease. Armed with grants and bigger microscopes, researchers began to test the impact of the known antioxidants.

As retold by the Harvard School of Public Health Nutrition Source, "Even before the results of the trials were in, the media, and the supplement and food industries began to hype the benefits of 'antioxidants.'" But the results of the trials were inconclusive, especially about the value of antioxidants delivered by manufactured supplements.

So go straight to the sources. As Harvard's educators observed, abundant evidence suggests that eating whole fruits, vegetables, and whole grains -- all rich in networks of antioxidants and their helper molecules -- provide protection against many of these scourges of aging.[233]

COCOA PUFFERY

The mesmerizing power of antioxidants is evident in the recent ascension of dark chocolate to health food status. Both Mars, Inc. and Hershey, the Ford and GM of the candy business, were quick to seize on new science which seems to prove, in the new vernacular of nutritionism, that cocoa is a great source of antioxidant flavonoids. Those nutrients have been linked to lower blood pressure and a reduced risk of death.

Cocoa has enjoyed a good reputation for centuries. Until recently, all it took was some oil and sugar to produce the extremely popular medicine known as chocolate. Dark chocolate, regardless of its name or marketing, has a larger share of cocoa bean solids, and therefore more of the nutrients associated with health benefits.

But chocolate bars are not tomatoes or broccoli, so watch out for the fats and carbs. Spend a little more for the bars with 70 percent cocoa, or just slip some unsweetened cocoa into your morning coffee and taste the achievement.

233: Yara.

THANK YOU BERRY MUCH

You'd think blueberries would make it onto any what-to-eat list just by virtue of being blue or round or cute or delicious. In the micronutrient age, blueberries have graduated from being a mere muffin ingredient. Today's blueberries are exalted as a repository of antioxidants trained to regulate cholesterol and prevent osteoporosis. Good to know. Good to eat.

But wait! Raspberry producers have their own research. Their tart and seedy berries have 10 times more antioxidants than tomatoes or broccoli, and some specific antioxidants that are found almost nowhere else. Okay, I'll have some of those, too.

Not so fast! According to a Pennsylvania researcher who considers himself "The World's Top Anti-Aging Specialist," the top dog among free radical killers is the chokeberry, followed by black currant and the elderberry.

Chokeberry juice is black and sour, concedes Dr. Dave Woynarowski. "I don't really care for it, so I take the capsules." [234] Okay, chokeberry loses on flavor and appeal, although it has been gaining advocates under the easier-to-swallow name of aronia.

The take-home message remains the same: Eat and enjoy a wide variety of foods and get all your important little molecules of this and that the old-fashioned, unprocessed way. Then work up a sweat in the garden.

234: "Blueberries Over-Hyped as Health Food." *PR Web*. October 9, 2005.

18

EDIBLES, A TO Z

For your consideration, members of the Academy: The Nominees for Best Foods, from A to Z. The items in the following list were suggested by several reliable sources, including "51 Health Foods You Can Say 'Yes' To," as compiled by nutritionists at Tufts University, Medford, Mass.

But first, a nutty sidebar too delicious to pass over: The athletic teams at Tufts University are called the Jumbos, in honor of the famous P.T. Barnum circus elephant by that name. The mammoth attraction perished spectacularly in 1885 when it was struck by a runaway locomotive. Never one to bury a top attraction, Barnum commissioned the world's largest taxidermy project and toured the world with the carcass for another four years before donating it to the university.

There it was proudly displayed until it was destroyed by an equally spectacular fire in 1975. As the smoke lifted, some of Jumbo's ashes were gathered into the first available container. A life-sized bronze sculpture of the iconic elephant was unveiled on campus in 2014. What remains of the original Jumbo can be found in the office of Tuft's Athletic Director, enshrined in a jar which originally contained 14 ounces of Peter Pan Crunchy Peanut Butter.

And so, with apologies to all the foods leapfrogged alphabetically by the peanut, here is the A to Z of healthy eating:

Acorn squash: Packed with vitamins, fiber, and potassium. Too squishy for you? Slice (unpeeled), bread and brown in a little olive oil.

Almonds: Packed with potassium, antioxidants, unsaturated fat, and calories. A healthy substitute for most fatty snack foods, and they might even improve your memory.

Apples: You know what they say. Is that why the doctor's wife eats them every day? They're all good. The red skins may have extra benefits. Peel not thy apple.

Apricots: Naturally flavored with vitamins A and C, as well as lycopene, which may reduce cancer risk in men.

Asparagus: The Vegetable of Kings is low in calories and high in vitamins and folic acid. Good warmed with dinner, or cold with a salad.

Bananas: The perfect potassium antidote for a typical day's sodium overload. Helps lower blood pressure, and reduce the risk of kidney stones and bone loss, or so they say. Also a good source of magnesium. They'll keep a little longer in the refrigerator, even though the peel looks less appealing. Personally, I find the organically grown varieties have more banana flavor.

Barley: Try cooking up the husky, whole-grain variety as a substitute for white rice. It's browner. It's better.

Beets: Like spinach, a super source of folate and betaine, and the stuff that imparts the famously red pigment fights cancer, at least in rats. Fresh and raw is best. Use a grater to make a salad tossed with olive oil and lemon juice.

Breakfast cereals: Just keep your eyes on the top shelf at the grocery. Most of that colorful crap positioned at eye level for children is devoid of whole grains, low in fiber and high in calories -- and shame on every media conglomerate that licenses their cartoon characters to sell that junk. Stick with the brands your grandmother knew: shredded wheat, Cheerios (plain, or new-fangled multi-grain), Grape Nuts, or bran flakes. Check for added salt, fats and sugars in many of the new concoctions claiming to be your healthy breakfast buddy. You're better off getting something simple with only a few ingredients, then adding fruit, nuts or honey at home.

Blueberries: Deserving of their healthy hype and suspiciously inexpensive much of the year. Couldn't growers pay those farm workers a lot more? Ditto for strawberries. In the off season, get them in frozen packages.

Bran flakes: There's a reason they're so close, alphabetically, to blueberries. A breakfast team made in heaven.

Broccoli: Most of us need to eat two or three times more of the dark green and leafy vegetable category. Broccoli, spinach and kale fill the bill. A pinch of sugar over steamed broccoli cuts the bitterness. At the Jennison Test Kitchen and Coffee Bar, we like to stir a little cream cheese into cooked spinach, and use a pressure cooker to quickly soften up a mess of kale.

Brown rice: Bran, germ and flavor are all included in the whole grain variety.

Brussel sprouts: Vitamin K makes it healthy. Halving, then roasting with lemon juice and a pinch of sugar makes it good.

Cabbage: Low in calories, filling and nutritious. Find a recipe for Asian-style slaw and rock your next office or family potluck. You will be admired and remembered, unlike whoever brought fake homemade cookies from the supermarket deli.

Garlic: Headed into the jungle? There is some evidence garlic may overpower the parasites that transmit malaria. But even when you are safe at home, those sulfur-based compounds that amuse or assault your nose may also suppress common bacteria and be good for your heart and fight cancer. Not exactly breaking news: Ancients in Italy, Greece, Egypt, India and China independently bestowed garlic with health food status. Just mash, mince and cook lightly to get the most flavor and benefit.

Canola oil: A healthy, versatile choice when olive oil seems inappropriate.

Cantaloupe: Packed with beta-carotene and vitamin C. Use your nose to pick out the best ones.

Carrots: A good, vitamin A-rich way to add some color to your plate.

Cauliflower: Why so white? Does it grow in a cave? Apparently not; it's packed with vitamin C.

Chicken breasts: Broiled, baked or grilled, a perfect protein entree.

Cranberries: Whole or juiced, the fruit has a singular reputation for discouraging urinary-tract infections, as well as gum disease. Now that dried cranberries have come down in price, we always have them on hand. Great on breakfast cereal, in muffins and -- trust me on this -- in a pecan pie all dressed up for Thanksgiving.

Eggs: Still recovering from years of bad press, but finally getting their due as an excellent protein source with all eight essential amino acids. A couple of golden yolks scrambled in the morning will stick with you a lot longer than a pale bagel. Although loaded with cholesterol, researchers now say only a small amount gets into the bloodstream. Saturated fats and trans fats from other sources are a bigger threat to your blood cholesterol levels than the healthy, unsaturated fat in eggs.

Kidney beans: Along with black, pinto, great northern and navy beans, they are packed with protein, fiber and other nutrients. Drain or rinse the canned beans to reduce salt content, or start with dried beans to feel like you're really cooking.

Mackerel: Not necessarily holy, but a go-to source for selenium, vitamin D and heart-healthy omega-3 fatty acids.

Oatmeal: MVP of the breakfast roster, oatmeal has real credibility as a filling and satisfying way to stay alert until the lunch hour while actually reducing bad cholesterol and high glycemic index. Start with "slow" whole oats -- it doesn't take much longer -- then add your own fruits and flavorings. I like apple butter, or a little maple syrup. Peaches, applesauce and walnuts aren't bad either. If you're really sweating the prep time, you can cook up a big pan of oats with some raisins on your day off, then refrigerate and reheat single servings.

Olive oil: Not just for food snobs, the famously healthy Italian immigrant should be a welcome guest in every American kitchen. Olive oil is a monounsaturated fat which can lower bad cholesterol in the blood. The virgin and extra-virgin varieties have the most antioxidants. Yes, some brands can be quite pricey, but remember, a quart lasts a lot longer than a gallon of milk. Big bottles offer some savings, but don't buy more than you can use before it goes bad. Use the less-expensive versions for cooking and fancier grades for side dishes and salads. Regardless, check the date on the bottle and get something less than a year old, then store it in a cool, dark place such as the box with your high school yearbooks, a sock drawer or, if more convenient, a kitchen cabinet.

Oranges: Liquid sunshine in an attractive, portable package, packed with vitamin C and potassium. I can slice and eat a whole one in less than two minutes.

Peaches: Sweet to eat, but only 40 calories. Just don't get the juice on your shirt -- makes a tough stain.

Peanut butter: Most of the fat in peanut butter is monounsaturated, making it a good protein alternative for most meat sandwiches. Good on anything from Wonder Bread to real whole wheat. Simple. Delicious.

Popcorn: Hey! It's a whole grain. An air popper makes it lean, for sure, but it's hard to get salt to stick without a little butter. Because you're going to buy the microwave bags anyway, look for the "natural" varieties with the least salt and oil. Eat enough of that "theater style" stuff and you won't live to see another movie.

Pork loin: This is the leanest cut of the wanna-be white meat. Three ounces provides a third of daily protein, and not much fat or calories. Pork producers say we no longer have to overcook pork to ensure safety. The USDA says cook to an internal temperature of 145 degrees. Until Health Canada completes its own reevaluation, its recommendation is 160 degrees. Regardless, a good meat thermometer will save you time and worry.

Prunes: Fiber, potassium, vitamins and other antioxidants. Why are you making that face? They are uniquely delicious.

Romaine lettuce: Along with Boston, Bibb and dark red or green leaf, a much better nutritional source than pale iceberg lettuce. Unless you just want to Make America Pale Again.

Red meat: Really? Sure, just don't spend more for "prime" cuts. They're loaded with fats. Choosing extra-lean cuts eliminates most of the fat concerns while treating yourself to protein that satisfies immediately and for several snack-avoiding hours to come. Outdoors types will also appreciate the low-fat alternatives of buffalo and venison. Can you spot the one that rhymes with the last name of your new, favorite author?

Salmon: Like mackerel, even the fat is good for you.

Sardines: More fishy goodness, and the bones contribute a little calcium. Read the label to find the least sodium and/or rinse and season to taste.

Shellfish: Clams, crayfish, crab, shrimp, scallops and oysters have all been unfairly branded with the scarlet "C" for cholesterol. Old food science: Shellfish are loaded with sterols, a group that includes cholesterol. New food science: Laboratory tests can now differentiate those sterols enough to know that shellfish are low in cholesterol, but rich in heart-healthy fats. Just skip the tub of dipping butter. Broiled, grilled or steamed, you'll savor the flavor of a heart-healthy protein.

Shredded wheat: Old school goodness with a good dose of magnesium.

Spinach: Not quite capable of producing instant biceps on a pop-eyed sailor, but it sure meets your MDR for dark green, leafy vegetables. And that kick of lutein might make it easier to read nutrition labels on your next trip to the food mart.

Strawberries: Very berry and a delicious delivery system for vitamins and fiber. They are an underpriced value during much of the year, partly because California farm workers must wait until 2022 for the same overtime pay rules already in place for all other employees.

Sweet potatoes: More vitamin C, calcium, manganese than their white in-laws, and much more beta-carotene. Sweet and good for you, but only if you eat 'em.

Tomatoes: Fruit or vegetable? Does it really matter? Vitamin C, lutein and lycopene up the health ante. Versatile in the kitchen and happy in the mouth, fresh tomatoes are the Number One reason to support your local farmers' market. Plus, you'll meet some interesting people.

Tuna: Great as a dinner entree and conveniently canned for a quick lunch. Go easy on the mayo and kick up the flavor with pickle relish, onions, olives, apple chunks and/or pecans.

Turkey breast: Enjoy the first meal of whole, fresh breast hot from the oven, then savor cold slices for sandwiches -- exquisitely void of the shredding and additives that make deli turkey a closer cousin to bologna.

Walnuts: Like almonds, a healthy alternative to most fatty snacks.

Watermelon: Low in calories, but a sweet source of vitamins and lycopene.

White fish: They're missing the omega-3 fatty acids of salmon, but flounder and cod are low-cal, high-protein goodness. Sure, fresh is best, and expensive. We're happy with frozen, store-brand value packs. The individually wrapped pieces thaw quickly in a big bowl of water. Baked, broiled, grilled or sauteed with a dash of oil on a non-stick skillet, they're idiot-proof and delicious, especially with a sprinkle of Old Bay seasoning or a good facsimile.

Whole-grain bread: The new food guidelines recommend that at least half of daily grains are whole-some. It doesn't matter how many health claims appear on the front of the package. If the first ingredient in the fine print isn't "whole grain," that bread is broken.

Whole-grain pasta: It's been several years since I've tried (and gagged on) said product, but my sources say there are new improved versions. I'll try it again, if you will.

Yogurt: The good stuff has protein, calcium, minerals and vitamins. The little flavored cartons are mostly overly processed desserts masquerading as health food. We mix the plainest of Greek yogurts with a little fruit, honey or cinnamon. A big spoonful straight from the carton is a great hunger buster between meals.

Zebra steak: Disappointing. The meat is all one color.

Zucchini: A respected and versatile vegetable.

19

LIQUID CALORIES

Awhile back, a committee of the American Medical Association reacted to a disturbing increase in the amount of sugar Americans were consuming. In particular, they noticed we were knocking back three full bottles of soft drinks -- per week!

That "while back" was 1942, and the cute and curvy bottles each held 6.5 ounces. Total: 19.5 ounces per week.[235]

How quaintly dated. How puritanically innocent. How spot on those same doctors were when they urged, 75 years ago, that we should just say no to sugars that are not already part of otherwise nutritious foods.

Today, of course, a soft drink container with less than 20 ounces is getting hard to find. Who's even looking when a 44-ounce pour at a convenience store or fast-food restaurant doesn't cost any more than a small cup? They're not being generous, you know. They're deflecting criticism over portion sizes by making it *your* call, *your fault* to super-size. And they know you'll probably pick a medium or large size (20 to 30 ounces) instead of the extra-large cup, so that you can still feel good about yourself while sipping up to 400 empty calories.

Since the days of the six-ounce pop bottle, food scientists have continued to lower the cost of refining or manufacturing sweeteners while finding more and more ways to punch those cheap sugars into thousands of products on every

---

235: Marion Nestle. *What to Eat*. North Point Press. 1994.

aisle of the supermarket. And each time we tried to execute an end-run around those high-calorie concerns, we were tackled by the latest study challenging the safety or our favorite diet sodas and artificial sweeteners.

No one is claiming 100 percent cause and effect, but there has to be more karma than coincidence in the fact that the nation's prevalence of obesity doubled during the same 24-year span when we also doubled down on drinking sweetened beverages.

One study attributes one-fifth of all weight gain among Americans over a 30-year period to sweetened beverages.[236] A series of studies have proven conclusively that among children and adults, there is a dependable correlation between sodas popped and pounds added. The only way to dodge the conclusion is to accept the spin favored by the soft drink makers: that for many Americans, soft drinks are just one measure of an unhealthy lifestyle stuffed with junk foods and not enough exercise.

ADDED SUGARS, BY THE GULP

On paper, it's easy to suggest that the calories enjoyed in a sweet soda or fruit-sweetened blend can be offset by skipping a like number of calories in some other part of the daily grazing routine. In the real world, sugary drinks contain nearly half (47 percent) of the added sugars Americans consume in a typical day. Sweetened drinks, however, lack the fats, solids and satiety that come in an equally sweet apple turnover or chocolate bar.

Broad studies of sugars and satiety have piled on the evidence. An article published by Yale researchers reviewed 88 other studies and concluded, plain and simple, that people who drink sweetened sodas get more calories in a typical day than people who don't. Soft drink intake also was associated with lower intakes of milk, calcium, and other nutrients and with an increased risk of several medical problems including diabetes. While they were at it, the Harvard review also documented that studies funded by the food industry reported significantly smaller effects than did non-industry-funded studies.[237]

236: Gail Woodward-Lopez and others. "To What Extent Have Sweetened Beverages Contributed to the Obesity Epidemic?" *Public Health Nutrition.* 2011

237: Vartanian, Schwartz, Brownell. ." Effects of Soft Drink consumption on Nutrition and Health: A Systematic Review and Meta-analysis". *American Journal of Public Health.*" 2007.

On a typical day, according to the Harvard School of Public Health, four out of five U.S. children and two out of three U.S. adults drink sugar-sweetened beverages, and lots of them. Teen boys average more than a quart of sugary drinks a day. Even adults trying to lose weight average more than two 12-ounce cans of sugary drinks a day. [238] [239] [240]

Harvard's health educators say that America's bulging thirst for sugar-water has clear correlations with obesity and Type 2 diabetes. "There is now strong evidence that sugary drinks have contributed mightily to the rapid growth of 'diabesity.' Women who have one or more servings of a sugary drink per day have nearly double the diabetes risk of women who rarely have sugary drinks, for example." [241]

Oh, it gets worse. Another study followed the health of nearly 90,000 women over two decades. It found that women who drank more than 2 servings of sugary beverage each day had a nearly 40 percent higher risk of heart disease compared to women who rarely drank sugary beverages. [242]

Across the globe, an estimated 184,450 deaths annually may been attributed to sugary drinks, according to a study published in 2015 by Tufts University's Friedman School of Nutrition Science & Policy in Boston. Of that total, 133,000 deaths were related to diabetes, 45,000 to cardiovascular disease and another 6,450 to cancer. [243]

Mexico and the U.S. ranked first and second in per capita deaths linked to wet sugar.

238: "Time to Focus on Healthier Drinks." *Harvard School of Public Health.* © 2011.

239: Bleich, Wang, Wang, Gortmaker. "Increasing Consumption of Sugar-Sweetened Beverages Among US Adults: 1988-1994 to 1999-2004." *American Journal of Clinical Nutrition.* 2009.

240: Wang, Bleich, Gortmaker. "Increasing Caloric Contribution From Sugar-Sweetened Beverages and 100% Fruit Juices among US Children and Adolescents, 1988-2004. *Pediatrics.* 2008; 121:e1604-14.

241: Schulze, Manson, Ludwig, Colditz, Stampfer, Willett, Hu. "Sugar-Sweetened Beverages, Weight Gain, and Incidence of Type 2 Diabetes in Young and Middle-Aged Women." *Journal of the American Medical Association.* 2004; 292:927-934.

242: Fung, Malik, Rexrode, Manson, Willett, Hu. "Sweetened Beverage Consumption and Risk of Coronary Heart Disease in Women." *American Journal of Clinical Nutrition.* 2009..

243: "Sugary Drinks Linked to High Death Tolls Worldwide." News release. *Tufts University.* June 29, 2015. Dariush Mozaffarian, M.D., dean of Tufts' Friedman School of Nutrition Science & Policy, was lead author of the study, which was published in the journal *Circulation* on the same date.

TEETH AND BONES

My family dentist used to tell me that sipping on a soft drink is like bathing your teeth in sugar. Unfortunately, he did not mean it was a shortcut to clean, sweet breath. The problem is that all those simple carbohydrates in sweetened beverages like to ferment in the mouth, producing acids which dissolve tooth enamel and put the teeth on a fast track to developing cavities. Although overall oral health has been improving for most Americans, a National Center for Health Statistics review has warned that tooth decay among young children was trending upward. The study's author blamed parents for overloading preschoolers with fruit snacks, juice boxes, candy and soft drinks.[244]

Other studies have suggested an association between soft drink consumption and reduced bone density, especially among women. One hypothesis puts most of the blame on cola-flavored drinks in particular because of their higher phosphoric acid content. That acid may displace calcium in the bones, thereby reducing bone density and contributing to osteoporosis. Or this may just be a another case of soft drinks being part of a lazy diet that doesn't include enough calcium-rich foods.[245]

Hey, guys! Here's one just for you. Gout. Most common in men aged 40 and over, gout is caused by excess uric acid in the blood. Too much of the stuff, and acid crystals form around bone joints, causing painful swelling. Gout is the most common inflammatory arthritis in men. Incidents of gout in the U.S. have doubled over the last few decades, according to a U.S.-Canadian research team that went looking for a culprit. Analyzing the food histories of 46,000 men over 40 years, they found a suspicious link, not only with soft drinks, but with fructose-rich juices and fruits, such as apples and oranges. Men who had two or more sweet drinks per day had an 85 percent higher risk for gout than men who drank less than one per month.[246]

HIGH-FRUCTOSE CORN SYRUP

Unrelated or coincidence? The rapid increase in overweight and obese Americans closely dovetails with the rise of cheap high-fructose corn syrup

---

244: "Tooth Decay On the Rise for Kids." *Associated Press*, as published in *USA Today*. April 30, 2007.
245: R.P Heaney and R. Rafferty. "Carbonated Beverages and Urinary Calcium Excretion." *American Journal of Clinical Nutrition*. September 2001.
246: Hyon K. Choi and Gary Curhan, "Soft Drinks, Fructose Consumption, And The Risk of Gout In Men: Prospective Cohort Study." *BMJ.com*. January 2008.

(HFCS) as the sweetener of choice for the biggest food processors.

The idea that high-fructose corn syrup may have a particular link to weight was raised in a 2004 research paper, then gained traction in 2005 when a group of hungry lab mice attended a party hosted by researchers at the University of Cincinnati. The menu included solid food and water for the control group. For the other rodents, solid food was paired with either a diet soft drink, a drink sweetened with sucrose (table sugar) or a fructose-sweetened drink. Only the mice fed with fructose gained significant weight.

Co-author Matthias Tschöp, MD, said consuming fructose appears to affect metabolic rates in a way that favors fat storage. "We were surprised to see that mice actually ate less when exposed to fructose-sweetened beverages, and therefore didn't consume more overall calories," he said. "Nevertheless, they gained significantly more body fat within a few weeks."[247]

Results from an earlier study in humans found that several hormones involved in the regulation of body weight, including leptin, insulin, and ghrelin, do not respond to fructose as they do to other types of carbohydrates, such as glucose.

"Similar to dietary fat, fructose doesn't appear to fully trigger the hormonal systems involved in the long-term control of food intake and energy metabolism," said Dr. Peter Havel, one of Tschöp's coauthors.[248]

Subsequent research has produced a few fructose-friendly findings, but mostly added evidence that the body has a strong preference for glucose, which can be converted to energy by virtually every cell in the body. Fructose -- which your grandparents knew as fruit sugar and came only from actual fruit and in small amounts -- can only be transformed in the liver, and not very well. When there is too much fructose, the liver converts it to fat, not energy. Eventually, the buildup resembles the liver condition associated with alcoholics.

Virtually unknown before 1980, nonalcoholic fatty liver disease now affects 30 percent of adults in the United States and other developed countries, according to a Harvard Medical School publication. Just as revealing, the

---

247: "New Link Between Soft Drinks, Weight Gain." University of Cincinnati Health News. August 2005. The referenced study appeared in the July 2005 issue of *Obesity Research*.

248: Same as above.

Harvard report says, the condition is evident in at least 70 percent of the population who are obese or have diabetes.[249] Researchers are still looking for a reliable way to test individuals for susceptibility to fructose-related liver damage.

BORN-AGAIN CORN

The powerful lobbyists with the Corn Refiners Association have worked hard to position their product as a healthy, natural and inexpensive alternative to the table sugars made from cane and beets. The low cost of HFCS is unquestioned. And it's certainly more natural than most of the artificial sweeteners it competes with. But don't stick a tap into a corn stalk and expect to fill a bucket with HFCS.

The basic science for making HFCS was around in 1957, then scaled to mass production by the Japanese in the late 1960s. But HFCS didn't reach an escape velocity until it was fueled by politics and market forces in the mid-1970s. Responding to fast-climbing grocery prices, President Richard Nixon and his Secretary of Agriculture, Earl Butz, reversed several New Deal policies aimed at supporting farm prices by discouraging overproduction. Instead, Butz urged farmers to plant their fields from "fence row to fence row." Corn production soared; corn prices fell. Between 1970 and its peak in 1999, our consumption of HFCS increased by a factor of 125 times – from .3 pounds per person per year to 37.5 pounds per capita annually. The big jolt came in 1984 when major soft drink manufacturers in the U.S. switched from sucrose to HFCS. Per capita consumption of cane and beet sugar dropped simultaneously, but has stabilized at about 44 pounds.[250] Add it up and each of us is eating and drinking about 25 added teaspoons of sugar every day or nearly 80 pounds of added sugar per year.

As negative publicity about consumption of HFCS increased, food and drink marketers reverted to using cane and beet sugar in some products. New packaging did more than adjust the fine print for product ingredients. Shoppers couldn't miss the new labels touting "real sugar," "retro," "throwback" or, loud and clear, "No HFCS!"

249: "Abundance Of Fructose Not Good for the Liver, Heart." Harvard Medical School, *Harvard Heart Letter*. September, 2011.
250: Same as above.

U.S. corn refiners responded with an attempt to rebrand their product as simply "corn sugar." Cane and beet sugar producers said that was deceptive and confusing and went to court to block the change. About the same time, the Food and Drug Administration formally denied the request. By 2015, the bitter battle of the sweeteners ended with a secret, out-of-court settlement.

DIET DILEMMA

Nearly a third of soda drinkers have bypassed the sucrose vs. fructose furor altogether. Ever preoccupied with dieting and calorie counting, millions of Americans each day choose the glamorous, thirst-quenching and fun-filled lifestyle promised or implied by the packaging and promotion of diet beverages.

It took two generations to accomplish, but diet brands now hold four of the top 10 sales position in the U.S.: No. 3 Diet Coke, No. 7 Diet Pepsi, No. 9 Diet Mt. Dew and No. 10 Coke Zero.[251] But in just the last few years, diet drinks have lost their fizz.

Industry analyst John Kell says factors much bigger than brand allegiance have dogged the bottled beverage business: "The growth of the 'clean living' movement is changing the food and beverage industries with an impact not seen since the advent of mass-produced food." Even soft drink makers who defend the safety of artificial sweeteners concede those products have developed a "stigma" sufficient to lower sales of diet beverages by 8 percent over the last two years.

Not that anyone is going thirsty. Sales of bottled water have been increasing for at least five years, as much as 10 percent annually. The top brands of bottled water are produced by the same soft drink giants (e.g., Coke's Dasani and PepsiCo's Aquafina) which already knew a thing or two about consumers, convenience, and marketing.[252]

How times have changed. Pepsi-Cola, always an also-ran to Coca-Cola, was the first to take a chance on tarnishing its family name by introducing Diet Pepsi in 1964, but only after test marketing under a different name (Patio Diet

---

251: E.J. Schultz. "Pepsi Passes Diet Coke In Market Share As Artificial Sweeteners Fall Out of Favor." *Adage.com*. March 26, 2015.

252: John Kell. "Diet Soda Is In Big Trouble." *Fortune.com*. October 23, 2015.

Cola). Coke watched with interest, but also hedged by calling its first entrant Tab. In part because of its reluctance to suggest its classic brand was a good source of empty calories, Coke held out until 1982 before introducing Diet Coke. Each of the diet brands claimed to taste just like the originals but of course they didn't, and still don't. Even so, diet drinks are also cold, wet and oddly sweet, and became a tolerable low-guilt substitute for the real thing. And whoever gained weight drinking the stuff?

You, maybe.

HOW NOT TO FOOL YOUR BODY

There is mounting evidence that *consumption of diet drinks and artificial sweeteners is somehow associated with weight gain.* Yes, life can be cruel.

A Purdue University study published in 2008 involved 17 rat volunteers. Divided into two nearly equal groups (I don't know why they couldn't afford one more rat), the rodents were given their usual access to delicious rat chow. But first, they got a snack. Eight rats were served yogurt sweetened with real glucose; the other nine got yogurt sweetened only with no-calorie saccharin.

After just five weeks, it was clear the sugar-free yogurt group was eating more chow and taking in more total calories. They had 5 percent more body fat and gained 20 percent more weight than the rats with the sugar-sweetened appetizer.[253]

Unable to recruit a group of humans willing to subsist on daily meals of yogurt and chow, the University of Texas Health Science Center instead tracked the soft drink habits of 1,550 adults aged 25 to 64 for seven to eight years. A third of the 622 participants who were "normal" in weight at the start of the study went on to become overweight or obese.[254]

No surprise there. But among those drinking two or more sodas a day, the group indulging in caloric versions gained less weight: 47.2 percent became overweight or obese, compared to 57.1 percent among the diet soda martyrs. In a related study, the Texas team tracked the waistlines of 474 elderly participants

253: Denise Gellene. "Saccharin May Lead to Weight Gain." Los Angeles Times. February 11, 2008.
254: Daniel DeNoon. "Drink More Diet Soda, Gain More Weight?" *WebMD Medical News*. June 13, 2005.

for 10 years. Diet soft drink users showed a 70 percent greater increase in girth compared to non-diet drinkers.

Sharon P. Fowler, co-author of the Texas studies, says the correlation between diet drinks and weight gain may only be a marker. "One possible part of the explanation is that people who see they are beginning to gain weight may be more likely to switch from regular to diet soda" but continue to put on pounds for other reasons.

Okay. Maybe. But what about those lab rats? They weren't looking into a mirror and stressing about a getting ready for a class reunion. After their appetizer of sugar- or saccharin-sweetened yogurt, they just chowed down until they were satisfied. The saccharin yogurt was appetizing, all right, but the fake sweetener wasn't fooling their little rat bodies.

"If you offer your body something that tastes like a lot of calories, but it isn't there," Fowler says, "your body is alerted to the possibility that there is something there and it will search for the calories promised but not delivered."[255]

Other research is leading to the same conclusions and the expectation that other artificial sweeteners have the same subconscious, metabolism-skewing effect of intensifying the quest for the real calories and real satisfaction. And -- parents take note -- a separate study out of the University of Alberta showed the confusing calorie clues from "diet" foods appear to condition young rats to overeat.

FAKE SUGARS, REAL DANGERS?

In May 2000, after 23 years of study and debate, the U.S. National Toxicology Program dropped saccharin from its list of suspected cancer-causing chemicals. It would be the first of many artificial sweeteners brought in for questioning, then released back onto the streets after prosecutors failed to prove they were a danger to society.

Saccharin was another of science's accidental discoveries, dating all the way back to 1879. It became recognized as a cheap, patriotic and zero-calorie sweetener during the sugar rationing years of World Wars I and II. Post-war, the

---

255: DeNoon.

pink packets of Sweet'N Low began appearing in coffee shops. Diet Pepsi and Diet Coke were first introduced with saccharin. It was in chewing gum, breath mints, frozen desserts. It was everywhere.

Beginning in 1960, studies with lab rats showed that ridiculously high levels of saccharin intake were causing bladder cancers. Canada banned the stuff outright in 1977. The USDA had the same idea, but Congress stepped in and instead ordered the attachment of warning labels, pending further study. By 1991, the FDA quit calling for a ban. The warning labels were axed in 2001. A full pardon was granted in 2010. And consumers yawned because newer, sweeter – safer? -- artificial sugars had taken over the 'hood.

ASPARTAME

Long before saccharin was cleared from all wrongdoing (except for its spoiler role in school spelling tests), major food and drink makers grabbed the opportunity to switch to something -- anything! -- they could claim was healthier and better-tasting. Aspartame, discovered in 1965 by an employee of G.D. Searle and Co. who licked his fingers by accident while working on an anti-ulcer drug, fit the bill and went mainstream as soon as Diet Coke and Diet Pepsi made the switch in 1983 and 1984.

Even so, aspartame -- now marketed as NutraSweet and Equal and quietly added to thousands of brands of beverages and solids foods -- continues to court controversy. Once again, conflicting studies and politicized spins have dominated the discussion. Although aspartame may have been safe from the get-go, it didn't help that Searle was alleged to have falsified test data during the convoluted 1970s FDA approval process. It didn't help when the U.S. Attorney General charged with investigating the allegations quit the case and took a job with the law firm representing Searle. It didn't help that millions of people helped give birth to Fake News when their new internet access allowed them to recirculate an aspartame conspiracy theory attributed to a still-unknown "Nancy Markle."

The worldly web is still crowded with anti-aspartame screeds, anecdotally linking it to fibromyalgia, spasms, shooting pains, numbness in the legs, cramps, vertigo, dizziness, headaches, tinnitus, joint pain, depression, anxiety attacks, slurred speech, blurred vision, or memory loss.

Headaches and migraines are most often cited by aspartame avoiders, but the biggest concern -- the Big C -- deserves and gets the most scrutiny. The most recent and credible attack on aspartame as a carcinogen came in 2005 with a study from the European Ramazzini Foundation on Oncology and Environmental Sciences, based in Bologna, Italy.

Regulators in the U.S. and Europe were initially swayed by the research but continued to pick away at the mechanics of the study and its findings, which were based on giving the rats the equivalent of 8 to 2,083 cans of diet soda per day.

Some 200 studies had already vouched for the safety of aspartame. Then in 2006 came the results of a five-year study of 567,000 U.S. men and women age 50 to 69. Comparing aspartame users and abstainers, the comparison found no evidence of increased risk for cancers and brain tumors.

So! If you're drinking a gallon or so of diet sodas per day, I really don't want to get to know you anyway. The rest of us can take some solace in knowing the world's second most widely used artificial sweetener has been found safe for humans in more than 90 countries. One FDA official called it "one of the most thoroughly tested and studied food additives the agency has ever approved." Its safety record, he said is "clear cut."[256]

Aspartame is still off-limits to the small number of people with a disorder called phenylketonuria, or PKU. These folks have trouble metabolizing a specific amino acid found in aspartame. A related sweetener called neotame is missing that acid and considered safe for the PKU crowd.

NEWER (SAFER?) SWEETENERS

Other artificial and alternative sweeteners have been introduced in recent years and studied enough to get FDA approval, or not even submitted for review.

Widely used but seldom mentioned in the office break room is one called *acesulfame potassium*, or *Ace-K*. The FDA approved it as a tabletop sweetener in 1988, with Sunnet and Sweet One being the brands you may have heard of.

256: John Henkel. "Sugar Substitutes: Americans Opt for Sweetness and Lite." *FDA Consumer Magazine*. November–December 1999.

Since 1998, it has been cleared for use in beverages and since 2003 for most foods. You probably consume more than you know. It is often combined with aspartame for such staples as Coke Zero, Diet Mt. Dew, Diet Pepsi, several store brands of diet soda and some low-cal versions of ice cream, whipped toppings and flavored gelatin. Even if you look at the tiny list of ingredients on food labels, you're probably experiencing eye strain before getting to the acesulfame potassium. The FDA says the safety of Ace-K is backed by more than 90 studies. The apolitical, harder-to-please Center for Science in the Public Interest says some of the research was inconclusive and wants more testing. "Until then, try to avoid it," the group says in its posted advisories.

Sucralose, popularized under the Splenda brand, is 600 times sweeter than sugar and was originally marketed as being "made from sugar so it tastes like sugar." The slogan never sat well with real sugar processors or the makers of a competing no-calorie sweetener, Equal. Harvard scientists say the chemical changes used to produce non-caloric sucralose produce something that's "not actually sugar any longer."

In 2007, the makers of Splenda settled a lawsuit over its disputed slogan moments before a jury was expected to side with Equal. U.S. sugar producers continue to discredit all artificial sweeteners and focus on "potential health consequences."

Splenda sales have been strong, in part because it is safe for diabetics and sufficiently stable for baking. Even before expanding to soft drinks, Splenda surpassed aspartame-based Equal and NutraSweet and good ol' saccharin-based Sweet'N Low. There's even a half-sugar, half-Splenda blend for customers who are only half-concerned about what gets past their lips.

The FDA gave its full approval to sucralose in 1999. Originally, the Center for Science in the Public Interest said there was "no reason to suspect that sucralose causes any harm." But as new research came in, the consumer activists downgraded their recommendation from "safe" to "caution" and then, in February 2016, to "avoid." CSPI's "avoid" list also includes ace-K, aspartame and saccharin.

Color-blind shoppers will want to read the labels when shopping for Equal. The egalitarian brand now uses different hues to package four different combinations of two or more ingredients: aspartame, ace-K, lactose, dextrose, sucralose and/or saccharine. Why don't they just mix them all together and call it Not Sugar?

Polyols: There is another group of sweeteners with only about one fourth fewer calories than regular sugar, but they taste good and don't cause tooth decay. We're talking about sugar alcohols (or polyols) such as mannitol, sorbitol and xylitol. They're said to be made by attaching hydrogen atoms to sugar molecules one at a time, by tiny hands in tiny factories. I'm still researching that. For sure, you'll find polyols in chewing gum, mints, toothpaste and prepared desserts. They're considered safe, but eating large amounts can cause what the FDA gently calls a "laxative effect."

One big caution for dog owners: two or three sticks of gum with xylitol can be very dangerous, even fatal. So keep any Altoids, Trident, Orbit, Icebreakers or Stride out of the reach of curious canines.

Stevia: Tired of all the confusion and controversy surrounding newer alternative sweeteners? Then you're already tired of this rising star. Stevia starts innocently enough as a sweet-leaf herb native to the warmest regions of the Americas. It was used for centuries in Paraguay as a sweetener and medicinal tea. Like Elvis Presley, it had to be discovered and repackaged by a marketing professional to make it from the boonies to the big stage. In 1931, French chemists isolated its sweetest components, stevioside and rebaudioside, and declared them 250 times sweeter than sucrose.

It took another 40 years and mainstream worries about cyclamate and saccharin to spur commercial production and processing. A Japanese company took the lead and created broad acceptance in that nation for stevia-based sweeteners in food products and soft drinks. Since the 1980s, wider acceptance of stevia as a dietary supplement or food additive has followed in China, the Soviet Union, Australia, France, Switzerland, Brazil, Mexico and, of course, Paraguay.

Regulators in the United States, like their counterparts in Canada and the European Union, have been more cautious. Lab tests dosing male rats and female hamsters with large doses of stevia derivatives have raised some concerns about infertility. Stevia was banned as food additive in the U.S. in 1987, but partially reinstated in 1995 under the infinitely more lenient rules for dietary supplements.

Coca-Cola and Cargill teamed up to produce a stevia-derived blend called Truvia. PepsiCo hooked up with a subsidiary of Equal's maker, Merisant, to create their blend with the equally wholesome and healthy sounding name of PureVia. They piled desks at the FDA with studies proving their side of the safety debate.

In December 2008, as employees of the George W. Bush administration were boxing up coffee-makers and rolling up rugs on their way out of the White House, the FDA signed off on the industry's appeal to give the stevia component rebaudioside the all-important status of "generally recognized as safe."

The Center for Science in the Public Interest had asked the FDA to wait for more research, citing some studies which suggested a cancer link. CSPI said the FDA's "midnight decision" to approve rebaudioside on the eve of a Republican-to-Democratic transition suggested the approval was based more on lobbying efforts than science.

"It's crazy that companies can just hire a few consultants to bless their new ingredients and rush them to market without any opportunity for the FDA and the public to review all the safety evidence," said the group's executive director, Michael F. Jacobson[257]

With the controversy still fresh, Coke and Pepsi moved rather cautiously in rolling out new products, including some that were later withdrawn from the market. Most recently, the competitors have gone head-to-head with two cola products sweetened with a mixture of sugar and stevia extract. They are Coca-Cola Life and Pepsi True.

So, can we trust products named after truth and life itself?

Your call.

257: "Lab Tests Point to Problems With Trendy New Stevia Sweetener." *Center for Science in the Public Interest* news release. August 28, 2008.

20

HOMEFRONT

FEED A FAMILY, STARVE A SCOLD

"I can't stop crying at the thought I could lose my beautiful children forever. This is every family's worst nightmare and I feel like we're being victimized," said the mother of six children -- all of them substantially overweight.[258]

Her predicament dominated the British press for weeks after a social services agency gave her three months to get three of their six fattest kids to slim down, or risk having all the children removed from the home. The three kids who were targeted were: a boy, age 12, weighing 244 pounds; a girl, age 11, weighing 168 pounds; and another sister, age 3 at the time and weighing 56 pounds. Their mother, age 39, weighed 23 ½ stone as the Brits say, or 330 pounds.

The family might have escaped the scrutiny of the fat police if they had not asked for help for the three-year-old, who had developmental problems.

"The parents have weight problems, but the children are spotlessly clean," a family friend said. "Had they struggled in silence, they wouldn't be in this horrendous situation."[259] Clearly, this obese, dysfunctional, and distressed family does not meet our minimum goal of achieving a fat, smart happiness. It's

---

258: Mark Smith. "Parents Told To Put Their Six Obese Children On A Diet or Face Having Them Taken Into Care." *The Mirror.* (London, UK). March 24, 2008.
259: Smith.

an extreme example, but not an isolated one. In the U.S., there are an estimated 2 million severely obese kids, defined as being in the heaviest 1 percent of their peers, based on BMI measurements.

But more than 13 million of the nation's 74 million children are considered obese. According to the last report by the. U.S. Centers for Disease Control and Prevention:

- 13.9 percent of children aged 2 to 5 are obese.

- 18.4 percent of children aged 6 to 11 are obese.

- 20.6 percent of adolescents aged 12 to 19 are obese.[260]

Experts in medical ethics in the U.S. and Britain are struggling to create guidelines for if and when it is appropriate for state or local agencies to intervene in households where a child is becoming dangerously overweight.

It has been accepted for decades that intervention may be necessary in cases where kids are malnourished or denied necessary medical care because of parental neglect. The view that over-nourishment constitutes neglect is a relatively new one, but not surprising considering that in just two decades, the prevalence for overweight in U.S. children ages 6-11 has doubled, and for teenagers, tripled.

Why is this the business of public health agencies? Because overweight children are at a higher risk for cardiovascular disease, Type 2 diabetes, asthma and other respiratory problems. Also, sleep disorders, liver disease, early puberty or menarche, skin infections or self-destructive eating disorders. If that's not troubling to you on a humanitarian level, also consider that a good chunk of your tax dollars go to treating those health issues.

For obese children themselves, medical concerns are too abstract or distant to worry about. They have more pressing concerns, like the school and neighborhood bullies whose taunts and teasing reinforce their low self-esteem and feelings of isolation and depression.

In the most extreme cases of childhood obesity, the threshold for accusing

---

260: "Prevalence of Obesity Among Adult and Youth: United States, 2015-2016." *cdc.gov*. October 2017.

parents of medical neglect remains high, as it should be. Weight alone doesn't tip the scale. Instead, family physicians or public health officers will focus on the likelihood that specific conditions such as diabetes and high blood pressure may predict serious, irreversible harm. Parents who heed the "wake-up call" and commit to improvements to diet and exercise will get plenty of support from doctors and social workers.

The evolving rules for legal intervention will target parents who don't even try -- the "adults" who refuse the advice of medical professionals or even undermine their child's efforts to steer clear of the sugar reefs. And that is why a handful of states from California, New Mexico and Iowa to Indiana, Pennsylvania and New York have begun to carefully apply the criteria for medical neglect in cases of severe obesity.[261,262]

I apologize for all the gloom and doom. These extreme cases are rare, but the lessons should be a heads-up for all parents. You get it. Don't you?

Maybe not.

PARENTS IN DENIAL

Several small studies have shown consistently that many parents see their overweight and obese children as being at a normal weight. A majority of overweight children have the same misconception.

Parents should not accept childhood obesity as the new normal when it continues to perpetuate stigma, prejudice, discrimination and bullying based solely on weight. As empathetic as I am to the fat acceptance movement, it seems the best opportunity for parents, pediatricians, and policy-makers to reverse an international "obesity crisis" lies with the youngsters who are just learning lifelong eating and exercise habits.

"Obesity is not a cosmetic issue; it is a highly significant health issue," says Dr. David L. Katz of the Yale University School of Medicine. "Because of our societal views, including widespread bias against obesity, there is considerable

---

261: Lindsey Murtagh, JD, MPH, and David S. Ludwig, MD, PhD. "State Intervention in Life-Threatening Childhood Obesity." Commentary. *JAMA* 2011.
262: Viner, Russell "When Does Childhood Obesity Become A Child Protection Issue?" Analysis. *BMJ*. August 2010.

pressure for parents and children to deny it even when they see it." De-stigmatizing obesity, he says, will lead to acknowledging and then addressing weight-related health issues in children.[263]

Most overweight kids have at least one overweight parent. Even for adults who recognize their kids are growing up with jelly bellies, efforts to intervene may be hampered by feelings of responsibility and guilt. Other parents may be adequately concerned and motivated, but are afraid they'll push too hard and turn mealtimes into a cage match and elevate a minor weight issue into an eating disorder. Understandable.

A recent, in-your-face media campaign in Atlanta, Ga. showed just how touchy the subject is. In billboards and television ads, overweight kids talk about being bullied at school or being scared by a doctor's warning. "Stop sugarcoating it, Georgia," the ominous voice-over said. "Warning: Being fat takes the fun out of being a kid," a billboard bellowed.

The campaign, called *Strong4Life*, was put together by a children's hospital, the YMCA, Boys and Girls Clubs of Metro Atlanta and the Georgia Department of Public Health. Organizers said the campaign was needed to raise awareness of the health concerns and bring the community together to work on solutions.[264]

Kudos for trying to raise awareness and work on solutions. But most parents don't appreciate having a tough love message directed at their own kids via TV and billboards, especially when school bullies interpret the public hazing as permission to take their bullying to the next level.

Labeling a person of any age as obese -- especially a child or adolescent -- is disparaging and counterproductive, says Peggy Howell, spokeswoman for the National Association to Advance Fat Acceptance. She says the tone and message of the *Strong4Life* campaign was "extraordinarily harmful" to overweight kids. If the program's sponsors really wanted to help, they should create an advertising campaign that "encourages people of all sizes to eat healthy food, add movement to our lives and celebrate our differences."[265]

263: Steven Reinberg. "Many Parents Are Blind To Their Kids' Weight Problem." *HealthDay*. June 4, 2004.
264: Ryan Schill. "Strong4Life's 'Tough Love' Childhood Obesity Campaign Creates Controversy." *Juvenile Justice Information Exchange*. jjie.org. September 23, 2011.
265: Schill.

That's a difficult message to convey to adults. Never mind trying to convince your own kids that their tormentors are really just concerned about their insulin resistance. Even health professionals struggle with terminologies. The American Medical Association has debated about whether they should bluntly label a child as fat or obese, even if it makes the family angry, or stick with the Centers for Disease Control's softer term, "at risk of overweight." Hard-liners argued that it was better to risk a child's self-esteem than his or her health.

Many family physicians are reluctant to discuss weight with young patients. Some are afraid of angering parents. Others, if they're moving toward the Health At Every Size® mindset, find more constructive things to discuss. A majority ignore national guidelines to measure, weigh and calculate a BMI for all kids twice a year. In fact, there are doctors who are uneasy about their own weight and therefore unwilling -- like overweight parents -- to venture very far into the knotty realm of "Do as I say; not as I do."

What happens in a doctor's office once or twice a year may matter little. Surveys show kids get most of their health information from their mothers, just as they are more likely to pick up bad eating habits from their fathers. The blame game is easy to play and has no winners. We would all like teachers, coaches, friends and friends' parents to be more sensitive, supportive and helpful. But the first responsibility for practicing (not preaching) positive attitudes and health habits resides at the same address where the kitchen, TV room and backyard are located. All parents lead by example. The challenge is to improve the example on display. With just a modicum of focus, effort, and consistency, parents can usually divert a heavy child's focus on food, mirrors, and weigh-ins by gradually introducing new habits that are both fun and healthy.

DO THIS. DON'T DO THAT.

Parents are accustomed to communicating in terms of do's and don't's. In the spirit of "Do flush the toilet" and "Don't bother a skunk," I have plumbed the advice of experts which, I suppose, now includes me. Behold:

Do be consistent. Do be predictable. But don't be rigid. Don't be afraid to bend rules when the situation demands. For example, Halloween treats, Thanksgiving casseroles and Christmas cookies will magically appear every year, regardless of your calorie goals. Do pay attention to portion sizes and limit grazing, no matter what the event, be it a birthday or funeral. If it's not too late, start early. Pediatricians say critical lifetime habits for eating and activity are established before the last bib is washed. Do rely on experts for advice on infant and toddler nutrition, especially if your own waistline indicates your instincts are deep-fried and sugar high.

If it's not too late, start even earlier. Expectant mothers have the best chance to lead by example during pregnancy. Studies have shown that before birth and while nursing, moms who enjoy fruits and vegetables can pass on a lifetime preference for the good stuff to their kids. Do realize that kids who are plump at age two are more likely to be overweight or obese in childhood and as adults.

Do accept the fact that about half of all two-year-olds are picky eaters, and they may grow up to be picky eaters. Continue to make healthy options available and lead by example.

Do keep it simple. Toddlers tend to prefer foods that are kept separate, not mixed or mashed, because one ingredient can spoil the whole recipe. Put some effort into making a fun presentation.

Do avoid food fights you're not going to win. Instead, follow Cookie Monster's lead, and teach that all foods can be enjoyed, but some are Anytime Foods and others are Sometimes Foods. Don't use food for rewards or make it synonymous with love and acceptance. Hugs are for love. Food is for filling tummies and diapers.

Don't bring home big cakes or bags of candy. Instead of being available for all-day snacking and grazing, make sweets a rare and wonderful treat. Celebrate Fridays with the kids' favorite candy bar as an after-dinner dessert.

Do point out positive role models who are not thin. Talk about weight-based stereotypes and then point out the exceptions you know or see on TV. Teach that thick and thin are a poor measure of what is within. Do emphasize health and strength, rather than thinness, when discussing foods and portions. Boys and girls all like the idea of being stronger, running faster and playing longer. Do be positive in your reinforcement. Kids often respond to good advice if adults can let them forget who it came from. Stubborn brats. Sweet angels!

Do not be negative. You'll only succeed at adding to stress and stigma, and possibly contribute to weight gain or an eating disorder. Studies have shown a stern, combative approach is more likely to spawn overweight children. Being overly permissive will get the same, fat results. Be authoritative, not authoritarian. Bend. Don't snap. Give copies of this book to your fat friends so they can be smart, happy and authoritative.

Don't obsess about your own weight, eating and exercise. Recognize fat phobia and don't contribute to it. Kids who learn to equate fat with failure may starve themselves right into the hospital. They're kids. They don't have to lose many pounds to get sick. Try moving the ball forward by introducing healthier ingredients in family favorites. Ease into it or you'll get called for interference and take a 10-yard penalty.

DRINK THIS, NOT THAT.

Don't encourage fat children to drink diet sodas. As discussed earlier, the confusing clues about calorie content may encourage overeating in other ways. Instead of soft drinks and uber-sweetened bottled teas, make delicious iced tea and real fruit drinks. You'll save a lot on both money and calories.

Ice tea: Steep one family size or three small tea bags (we love Luzianne) into a pot of almost-boiling water for five minutes, then dissolve a fourth cup of sugar and add enough water to make two quarts. Serve cold. Compared to 160 calories in a 12-ounce soft drink, the home brew yields only 34 calories for the same amount.

Orange juice has more calories per ounce than soft drinks, although a "serving" is just eight ounces. Regardless, low-acid orange juice (from a carton or concentrate) mixed half-and-half with water and nicely chilled makes a refreshing, healthy alternative with 90 calories per 12 ounces, even less if you dilute it further. Just remember it's a replacement for soft drinks, not a legitimate serving of fruit.

BUT WAIT! THERE'S MORE!

Don't blame schools, television, video games or Micky D for your child's belly fat. The buck stops with the parents, grandparents, siblings and other caregivers who have the responsibility to lead by example.

Don't encourage or allow children to go on a weight-loss diet. As with adults, pounds should come off at the same pace they came on -- s l o w l y. One study put one group of kids on a closely supervised program of exercise and nutrition education, Yes, it worked, but researchers conceded it would be expensive or unrealistic for most families to maintain. Another group in the same study was put on a strict diet. Well, Ma'am, that part of the study had to be aborted. Too many drop-outs! Even kids know there is something crazy wrong with starving yourself.

Ever since Milton Berle, Soupy Sales and Mighty Mouse made TV a habit for families and kids, television has gotten non-stop blame for fertilizing a steady crop of couch potatoes. Today, with computers, smartphones and video games competing for eyeballs, the affliction is known as excessive screen time.

Try to schedule TV and computer time for *after* the kids have had a proper snack or a real meal. Watching TV with a bag of chips and a jug of sugar water in hand is what gave TV a bad name. Well, that and *The Jerry Springer Show*. To keep it simple, just don't allow eating in front of the TV.

Meanwhile, stay on the lookout for new ways to promote all manner of non-screen activities. Keep indoor and outdoor motion in mind when gift shopping for birthdays, holidays, a full moon, a clean bathtub or any equally lame excuse to break a sweat and have some fun.

I don't think playing with Barbies or toy soldiers spawned any more indoor exercise than smart phones back when I was a rugrat. But we did work up a sweat close to home with an inexpensive basketball, football or softball. And don't forget Wiffle Ball, with its yellow, plastic bat and a white slotted ball. It's pitch perfect for any yard and comes with no broken windows.

Help kids find solo and pairs activities they can enjoy for life. Dodgeball and soccer are great for P.E. class, and team sports are valuable for many reasons. But when kids move on to college, work and adulthood, they shouldn't need to exchange more than one or two text messages to organize a racquetball match, bike trek, golf outing or Frisbee toss.

Do get a dog. Don't get a little dog that gets ample exercise jumping onto the couch 30 times a day. Get a big dog that deserves and expects a good, long walk twice a day. Make it a habit. Don't beg off just because the weather isn't perfect. Your dog won't be embarrassed at all by your sweat-stained sun visor, overstuffed winter coat or a SpongeBob SquarePants umbrella.

Do provide a healthy, substantial snack after school and a maybe a little something between supper and bedtime. Through example, not preaching, teach that snacking on munchies and sugar water throughout the day adds up to as many calories as a good meal, with none of the nutrition and feel-good fullness. Keep a bowl of fresh fruit in plain sight and cut-up vegetables ready to grab from the refrigerator.

Don't nag a child about weight. A child is not suddenly responsible for his or her weight. It's a family matter, to be addressed in a stigma-free, positive way. Do talk about strength, speed and agility. I repeat this because it's the most important maxim in the chapter.

Do make every effort to get the family together at one table for dinner.

Do prepare a healthy supper without making a big deal about it. Don't ask the kids what they want, unless it's a choice between two healthy options. They can decide not to eat it, but offer something leaner than ice cream when they come back hungry an hour later.

Portion sizes matter a lot. With the exception of vegetables, kids and adults are likely to eat more food when there is more to look at. (Studies among moviegoers with tubs of fresh and stale popcorn have shown large portions influence overeating more than taste. Perhaps you were in that study and didn't know it?) At home, use small plates. Obviously, a full small plate is going to look more satisfying than a big plate with the same sized portions. Do not put serving dishes on the table unless you're having special guests. Otherwise, just serve each plate in the kitchen with modest portions and immediately put any leftovers in the refrigerator to chill. Whether you eat them later or end up throwing them out will have no impact on starving kids around the globe. Make a cash donation for that.

Bulk up your foods, not yourself. A pasta salad is just lazy carbs unless you load it up with black beans, broccoli, tomatoes, carrots, cucumbers or zucchini. For the most part, avoid white foods, especially sugar, white rice, white flour, school paste and white, lead-based paint. The complex carbohydrates in whole grains are more satisfying and better for you.

Dining out or take-home meals are inevitable, and should be fun for everyone, but not the default routine for busy days. It's no coincidence that restaurants are switching to larger plates and chairs. Pay close attention to portions sizes and beverage choices. Milk is good; water is free. In our neck of the woods, sweet iced tea is often sweeter than colas. We ask them to mix it half-and-half with unsweetened tea, or we do it ourselves when it's self-service.

Do not insist that kids clean up their plates. Do not eat their leftovers yourself just because it cost too dang much to waste. Lay a napkin over an unfinished meal to signal a job well done, or bring home some leftovers if they're worth the space in your fridge. It might make a decent breakfast or lunch for someone tomorrow. Adults can set a good example and save some real money by sharing a plate wherever portions are ridiculously large, and that's just about everywhere these days. Share your savings with an extra-nice tip for your server.

Avoid the all-you-can-eat buffet. When coerced to participate by in-laws or co-workers, take plenty of time to savor soup and salad before inspecting the main pig trough. Eat smart so that you're not sorry and sleepy an hour later.

Do not teach your kids by example that a yo-yo cycle of starving and bingeing is normal. Don't be the face of guilt and denial. Children, especially girls, will learn to relax and enjoy healthy eating if that's what they see across the table.

Do make time for everyone to have a good breakfast. Protein, fruit and whole grains will help students (and adults) have a steady, alert morning. Sugars and lazy carbs are a good recipe for nodding off an hour later. "A good breakfast" doesn't mean bacon and pancakes every day. Most days, stick with some healthy protein, whole grain carbs and fresh fruit.

Do be attentive to internal signs of real hunger. Do be suspicious of external cues, including large portions. Find food. Don't let it find you. There's a difference between actually craving chocolate when there is none in sight, and strolling past a bowl of chocolates and thinking "Hey, get 'em before they're gone." Do get the blues. Not many of your favorite foods are blue. There's a reason for that. For many people, the color of skies and seas is an appetite suppressant. So try a blue tablecloth and blue plates and see if you're ready to leave the table sooner.

Instead of butter, cream, and sugar, kick up the flavor on worn-out favorites with zesty Cajun or Southwest spices, some of which will actually contribute to calorie burning.

If you want to get fun and fancy, serve meals one course at a time, but only if you start with soup, salad, or vegetables. You'll probably be getting full by the time the meat comes around. And dessert -- who cares? Too full.

Nuts to you and your kids. Low-salt cashews and almonds are dense, satisfying and nutritious. But don't go overboard. Most nuts, except almonds, are high in fats.

Get nosy. Just sniffing many foods is enough to trick the brain into curbing appetite.

Don't assume that by overeating or stretching a meal out over a long time that you'll compensate later by eating less. Studies show it just isn't so.

Make regular physical activity a part of daily routines. Nothing clears the head and stomach like a walk after dinner. Shoot some hoops, kick a soccer ball around the yard or gang up on the kids in a bruising game of dodgeball. When fall arrives and the days are shorter and the TV schedule more tempting, announce that you will DVR some family favorites for "viewing later." Because there's already too much on TV to consume, you won't get around to the saved episodes anyway.

Don't force kids to eat a lot of something new. Ask them to try two bites before deciding if it's thumbs up or tongue out.

Don't ban certain foods. That just makes them more attractive, the better to hide under a bed or gorge on away from home.

Make healthy snacks easy to find when kids are prowling. Endeavor to usually be out of salty, sugary fake foods. Instead, have sliced cheese, fruits and vegetables ready to grab from the frig. Encourage tablecentric snacking, as opposed to grazing on the couch,

Make time, on the weekends if necessary, to prepare healthy sack lunches for the week ahead. Those prepackaged lunch kits at the supermarket are super-soaked with salt, fat and unpronounceables. Handy, yes, but so is a thumb in the eye.

When kids tag along on trips to the grocery, make it a fun, learning experience. Show them how to compare nutrition labels, then make a game out of finding the ones with the least added salt, fat and sugar.

Don't go overboard with fat phobias. Kids need a healthy diet with about 30 percent of total calories coming from fats, preferably unsaturated plant sources. Everyone needs essential fatty acids and fat-soluble vitamins.

Get the kids a pedometer and let the natural competitive nature of siblings take over.

Be consistent with the who, what, and when of occasional treats. If Saturday is Pepsi and pizza night, then six other days are not Pepsi and pizza night.

For many people, stepping regularly onto a bathroom scale can be stressful and counterproductive, especially when the results aren't as expected. Still, it might be helpful to pack one for college-bound kids, who typically gain 15 pounds during their first semester away from home. A weekly weigh-in is a good reminder that with independence (and a meal ticket) comes great responsibility.

FAT CATS, FLUFFY DOGS

Empty-nesters who need someone to feed and care for eventually find that cats and dogs make a pretty good substitute for missing children. For starters, they don't ask for money, wreck your car, or come home drunk with a new piercing. However, they are more likely to shred furniture and pee on the floor. Cats and dogs are easy to spoil with toys and treats and table scraps. Stick with the toys and games. About one in four cats and dogs are overweight, defined as weighing 15 percent more than the optimum weight for its breed and sex. Quite a few are obese, defined as 30 percent over optimum. And, just as they are with children, pet-owners are notorious for not recognizing weight problems.

Overweight pets are extra cute if you're not concerned about increasing the likelihood of kidney stones, shortness of breath, arthritis, hip dysplasia, cancers and a shorter lifetime. Treatments and surgery are very expensive. Like, week-at-the-beach expensive.

Aside from skimping on exercise, giving people-food to pets is the biggest no-no. It's easy to lose a sense of scale. But giving a 20-pound dog one oatmeal cookie may be the caloric equivalent of a 5-foot-4 adult eating a hamburger and a chocolate bar. A hot dog and bun for the same dog equals three burgers and two candy bars for his human. Kitty wants a piece of cheese? No doubt, but one ounce of cheddar to a 10-pound cat translates to 3 1/2 burgers and four chocolate bars, according to graphic reminders posted in our veterinarian's waiting room.

So just don't teach pets to expect table treats. Stick with ample water and carefully measured amounts of pet food while keeping track of weight changes recorded during visits to the vet.

IN THE ARENA: HOW THE SHOPPING GAME IS PLAYED

When you push a cart down a grocery aisle, it's just you and your resolve versus millions of dollars in food science and literally tons of added salt and sugars. You're up against merchandising muscle spanning test groups, seductive advertising, colorful packaging and deliberate shelf positioning. You try to be mindful of ingredients, only to drive yourself blind and crazy trying to read nutrition labels and their tiny ALL-CAP LIST OF FIVE-SYLLABLE CHEMISTRY BOOK INGREDIENTS.

You can bypass much of the fine print simply by loading your cart with fresh fruits, vegetables, grains and protein. No labels, no ingredients -- just real food. Shopping for meats and dairy products in a little more complicated, but mainly requires some attention to the amount of fats included. Head back to the checkout area via the frozen vegetable aisle. Avoid the creamy, saucy and seasoned vegetable mixes which just add fats and salt.

Stay out of the middle of the store as much as possible. That's where the heavily processed foods wait to tempt you with their bleached flour, corn sugars and trans fats. Yes, there will be times you have to go on patrol for staples such as spices, corn meal, peanut butter, and olive oil. Just focus on your mission, with grocery list in hand and blinders to all that other stuff screaming "Eat me, I'm fun!" You'll also save a lot of money.

You don't see apples and bananas making health claims. Beware of foods that do, and processed products that take advantage of being "part of a healthy food group." Some brands of granola have more added sugar or fats than the fiberless puffs pitched to kids. Yogurt and nuts are healthy in moderation, but the heavily flavored or sweetened versions are just snack foods and desserts masquerading as fitness foods.

The larger the health claims on the front, the more you need to inspect the actual ingredients. Labels that say "All Natural" or "Made with Whole Grains" are increasingly common and all designed to encourage your guilt-free purchase. The FDA and USDA attempt to standardize and regulate such phrases but often succumb to constant pressure from food industry lobbyists to accept definitions which don't have much to do with everyday English.

Thus, some "All Natural" tomato sauce is made from reconstituted tomato paste shipped cross-country in 55-gallon drums. "All Natural" deli meats are injected with water and additives you'd never use at home. Factory-rendered high fructose corn syrup is just another "All Natural" ingredient these days. That loaf of bread or cereal wants you to know it was "Made with Whole Grains," so you won't notice it's mostly made with refined or bleached flour and dark brown coloring. If the label says "Made with Real Fruit," you might see a picture of strawberries or grapes on the front. On the back, you'll learn the filling is mostly sugar, pear juice concentrate, food colors and a molecule or two of "natural or artificial flavoring."

And look how many fun foods and drinks are now a "great source of fiber!" Okay, but what kind of fiber? Natural, intact fiber like that found in whole grains, fruits, vegetables and beans are known to have real health benefits. But processed, hype-driven foods are more likely to base their claims on the addition of purified powders and isolated fibers that occur naturally only in laboratories.

There will be times when cravings or convenience dictate that some processed foods and pantry staples will fall into your cart and go unnoticed until you get home. The food giants want your business whether you're picky or not, so look for differences even within the same brand. Some Rice-A-Roni has whole grains; some has less salt. Kraft Deluxe Macaroni and Cheese Dinner made with 2 percent milk cheese has a little more salt but less than half the saturated fat of its "original flavor." Dannon All Natural Low Fat Vanilla yogurt has as much sugar as some candy bars. Try Dannon Light & Fit or plain Greek versions instead.

You'll find an equally wacko range of salt, fat and sugar by comparing the labels on deli meats, hot dogs, sausage, bread, rolls, pastries, tortillas, pancake mixes, hot and cold breakfast cereals, condiments, pasta sauce, salsa, frozen entrees, ice cream and "energy" foods.

Salt and sugar are the cheapest ingredients available to processors. You will pay a little more for the healthier options. But have you priced liposuction or gastric banding lately? Just remember that pounds go on a lot cheaper than they come off.

Foods labeled "organic" have come to earn a surprising amount of display space in recent years partly, I think, because "all natural" had become so overused and abused. Fresh fruits and vegetables which earn the FDA's organic label are grown without the chemical fertilizers or pesticides which may leave a residue on non-organic apples, bell peppers, spinach, celery, grapes, peaches, or berries.

Organically produced foods are grown in richer soils and probably have a higher mineral content and perhaps more vitamins. The "organic" label actually means the item was at least 95 percent organically produced. If that's not good enough (And how can we really know?) seek out the "100 percent organic" sticker. But if you trust the USDA to closely police this frontier land as much as you trust the guy across the street to return your hedge clippers, get to know a real farmer who grows real food.

FUNCTION JUNCTION

"Vitamin-enriched" this and that have been popping up on grocery shelves for as long as guilt has been marketed to mothers. Today, the category of "functional foods and beverages" is more rambunctious than it's been since doctors wrote out millions of prescriptions for medicinal whiskey during Prohibition. Cereals, energy drinks, power bars and vitamin water are quickly replacing sales of chips and soft drinks for a population that pays lip service to nutrition but can't make time to peel an orange.

Japan is paving the way with hundreds of medicated foods said to boost immunity, tame allergies or fight disease. In the U.S., testing, definitions, and regulation are still in their infancy. So far, the FDA is mostly looking the other way, just as it always has done with the massive vitamin and supplements industry.

We had pretty good reasons generations ago for adding iodine to salt and fluoride to tap water. Perhaps the next great leap forward will be to put vitamins and protein in donuts and beer. Analogous or not, I'm just suggesting your next trip to the grocery would be a good time to think about the differences between actual whole foods and manufactured "functional foods." And how much of each you want to take home to your family.

21

EXERCISE AND SLEEP

merica, you're pretty fat and lazy!

I half apologize for saying that, not because it's rude and unhelpful, but because it's only half true.

Yes, we're collectively fatter. That's obvious. Well, not you in particular. You look great. But that persistent harping about adults and children melting into a fat tub of goo on the couch in front of the flat screen? That's mostly mouth exercise by the companies selling memberships to health clubs where skinny singles and flabby divorcees dream of making a love connection. Mostly, they will leave alone, tired, sore, and very hungry.

In a nation where a solid majority still equate personal worth with hard work and responsibility, it's no surprise that so much blame for obesity is pinned on weak minds and bodies at rest, rather than a surplus of cheap calories and the marketing muscle behind them. But the mantra that activity levels are directly related to body weight is relatively new.

As late as the 1950s, overweight patients were routinely advised to get more bed rest, not more exercise. Scientists had learned to calculate the miniscule number of calories burned through exertion -- about 3 calories for a heavy man to climb one flight of stairs. Besides, exercise for its own sake was a hard sell in the early days of Philco televisions, Chevy convertibles, and Otis elevators.

The turning point came with a little research and a lot of crusading by nutritionist Jean Mayer, according to science writer Gary Taubes. Taubes is the guy who defiantly challenged firmly entrenched Conventional Wisdom about the dangers of dietary fat in his 2002 *New York Times Magazine* piece, "What If It's All Been a Big Fat Lie?"

Mayer, a nutritionist at Tufts University, was convinced that exercise did not increase hunger and based his conclusions on two, and only two, of his own studies. By 1959, the *New York Times* was crediting Mayer with overturning the previous Conventional Wisdom that exercise played little role in weight control. According to Taubes, "It was Mayer who pioneered the now-ubiquitous practice of implicating sedentary living as the 'most important factor' leading to obesity and the chronic diseases that accompany it."[266]

In the following years, health writers paid more attention to Mayer and to each other than to newer studies and dissenting views. And so by the late 1970s, America was in the midst of a "fitness explosion." *Rolling Stone* chronicled and romanticized the rise of L.A. health clubs as the hook-up successor to singles bars, setting up the 1985 film "Perfect" starring the very hard bodies of John Travolta and Jamie Lee Curtis.

If the movie had been more accurate, the stars' sweaty workouts would have ended with fewer pushups in the bedroom and more frozen yogurt on the patio. There was plenty of concurrent research detailing the body's stubborn preference for homeostasis and the powerful hormones which insist on storing surplus calories as fat. (See Chapter 9, "Metabolism.")

"This research has never been controversial. It's simply been considered irrelevant by authorities," Taubes wrote in a 2007 *New York Magazine* article in which he deconstructed Stairmaster science as effectively as he had denounced the emphasis on reducing dietary fats five years earlier.[267] More recently, a group of researchers used national food supply data from the 1970s and early 2000s to calculate how many calories Americans were actually producing and eating. They also devised formulas to account for metabolism, thermodynamics, disease and farm production during the same time span in order to predict the resulting weight gain, and finally, compare that to actual weight gain.

266: Gary Taubes. "The Scientist and the Stairmaster." New York Magazine. September 24, 2007.
267: Taubes.

The math was over my head, but the conclusion was clear to Boyd Swinburn, M.D., lead author of the study: "Weight gain in the American population seems to be virtually all explained by eating more calories. It appears that changes in physical activity played a minimal role." [268]

Among children, the predicted weight gain perfectly matched that actual increase -- about 9 pounds -- suggesting that increases in caloric intake alone explained it. Adults actually gained less than was predicted -- about 19 pounds instead of 24 -- suggesting Americans actually became *more active* during the 30-year span of the study.

Physical activity is good for everyone. The health benefits are numerous and well documented. It's just that weight loss is something our bodies are hardwired to resist. You're alive today because all of your ancestors since the dawn of mankind attached a subconscious, primordial significance to storing fat that was far greater than any conscious effort to fit into a sexier boar's hide.

TIME magazine rankled America when it selected Russia's hard-nosed President Vladimir Putin as its Man of the Year in 2007. That was just a prank to finish a slow news year compared to the poke in the eye delivered by a 2009 cover story. The doomsday headline was: "Why Exercise Won't Make You Thin."

Digging into his worst fears, writer John Cloud found he wasn't the only one to spend dizzying hours on treadmills and stair-climbers week after week, year after year, only to maintain the same weight and a flap of flab still keeping his belt buckle in the shade. It wouldn't be fair, he thought, that a muffin, a fruit smoothie or cool blast of energy drink after all that sweating would negate the hundreds of calories burned at a virtual Altar of the Elevated Pulse.[269]

But the anecdotal and scientific evidence Cloud pursued with equal diligence was uniformly discouraging. Eric Ravussin, a metabolism and exercise researcher at Louisiana State University, summarized the latest research: "In general, for weight loss, exercise is pretty useless." [270]

He was reacting to a 2008 study by an LSU colleague and others which began with the recruitment of 411 sedentary, overweight or obese

268: Kristina Flore. "ECO (European Congress on Obesity): Obesity Blamed on Overeating, Not Inactivity." *MedPageToday.com*. May 28, 2009.
269: John Cloud. "Why Exercise Won't Make You Thin." *Time*. August 29, 2009.
270: Cloud.

postmenopausal women. They were divided into four groups, three of which were assigned a personal trainer to work them for either 72, 136 or 194 minutes per week, for six months. (The time intervals seem weird, but were carefully constructed to burn so many calories per pound per week.)

All the women, including the no-exercise control group, were told to maintain their usual eating and daily activity patterns.

At the six-month weigh-in, even the control group had lost a few pounds -- probably because filling out regular questionnaires made them more conscious of their calorie intake. (Try it yourself. It quickly becomes easier to not eat something if you have to write it down.) But the ladies with the trainers did not lose significantly more weight. Some even gained as much as 10 pounds. The mid-level exercise group lost the most weight -- about 4.6 pounds, on average. But the high-intensity group dropped only a few ounces more than the low-intensity group, 3.3 pounds versus 3.1 pounds.[271]

As in similar studies, the disappointing discrepancy between predicted and actual weight loss increased with the amount of exercise. While the women in the mid-intensity workout group got a good return on their sweat investment, the group getting 194 minutes per week got cheated at the weigh-in. Would you want to be the one to tell them most fitness advocates recommend 200 to 300 minutes of exercise per week?

The researchers explain the disappointing results by the very human trait for caloric compensation. The well-exercised women in the study either rewarded themselves for their grueling workout with a fast carbohydrate treat, or dialed back other physical activities, or some combination of the two.

Sometimes math sucks. The health club hero, for example, may climb the stair machine for a half-hour (- 360 calories), then head back home or to the office, stopping along the way for a much-deserved large cafe au lait (+375 calories).

271: Timothy S Church and others. "Changes in Weight, Waist Circumference and Compensatory Responses with Different Doses of Exercise Among Sedentary, Overweight, Postmenopausal Women." *www.plosone.org*. February 2009..

HERE TODAY. HERE TOMORROW.

As a means to weight loss, the heavy exercise tracked in the study was largely a failure. But women will be pleased to know the 411 females in the study did experience a "significant reduction in waist circumference." The belly-tightening was almost coincidental, however. The data showed only 11.6 percent of the waist loss correlated with actual weight loss.[272]

The good news / bad news about exercise is that it helps individuals *maintain* their present weight. Sequence is everything. Remember, your body will fight today to keep your weight the same as it was the day before. Exercise just makes the influence of homeostasis more powerful, especially for women.

It is only after a substantial weight loss achieved through calorie reduction that exercise becomes a friendly force, as confirmed by studies within the National Weight Control Registry.

The ongoing research tracks the weight and health habits of some 10,000 Americans who have lost at least 30 pounds and kept it off at least a year. On average, the participants (about 80 percent female) have lost 70 pounds and maintained their lower weight 5 1/2 years. Regular follow-ups have shown that 90 percent of the members who have maintained a weight loss also stuck with a regular fitness schedule.

In this study and others, "you see over and over that exercise is one constant among people who've maintained their weight loss," says Barry Braun, a University of Massachusetts kinesiologist.[273]

Again, exercise helps a person *maintain* their present weight, not reach a lower one.

TAKE IT TO HEART. EXERCISE STILL MATTERS.

I can hear many of you weight-hating gym rats screaming sentiments falling within the range of "This book is a health hazard!" to "Now you tell me!"

Chill.

272: Church.
273: Gretchen Reynolds. "Weighing the Evidence on Exercise." *The New York Times.* April 16, 2010.

It was all worthwhile.

Let's just take body weight out of the picture altogether. Instead, please look to these four important benefits of exercise, as smartly suggested by Go4Life, an exercise and physical activity campaign from the National Institutes of Health:

- *Endurance.* Exercises like brisk walking, dancing, or hiking improve the health of your heart, lungs, and circulatory system. Extra movement make it easier to tackle routine activities such as climbing three flights of stairs, mowing the lawn, or pushing your ex's junk to the curb.

- *Strength.* Strength training—like lifting weights or using resistance bands—can increase muscle strength and help with everyday activities like carrying bags of cat litter or garden soil.

- *Balance.* Balance exercises, such as standing on one leg or doing tai chi, can make it easier to walk on uneven surfaces and help prevent falls.

- *Flexibility.* Stretching exercises can help your body stay flexible. They give you more freedom of movement for daily activities, such as bending to tie your shoes or looking over your shoulder as you back out of the driveway or make an ATM withdrawal.

Is that not motivation enough? Don't you want to be flexible, balanced, strong, enduring, fat, smart and happy? Let's make it even simpler. Exercise just makes you feel better and sleep better.

Let's engage in some moderate activity right now with a brisk review of the latest findings about the benefits and myths surrounding exercise:

Now that most researchers agree that many of us have a genetic predisposition to obesity, one group reviewed 45 studies involving 218,166 adults and found that being physically active reduced the negative aspects of obesity by an average of 27 percent, suggesting that even genetic influences can be offset with a little grunt work.[274]

Obese women can improve their health without dieting by changing their eating habits and exercising more. A study at Leeds Metropolitan University

274: Jeannine Stein. "Exercise Could Counter the Effects of the 'Obesity Gene'" *latimes.com* November 1, 2011.

in England taught a group of women how to read food labels and prepare nutritious meals. After a year of that, with four hours of exercise per week, the women lost only a few pounds, but showed improvements in blood pressure, heart rates and cholesterol levels. And they were less stressed.[275]

Calorie reduction alone does not reduce the size of fat cells in the belly, but exercise does, according to a five-year Wake Forest University study. That's important because the size of the subcutaneous fat cells just under the skin is a good predictor of Type 2 diabetes. A diet-alone subgroup in the study had no change in the size of abdominal fat cells, but two groups burning about 400 calories per week through treadmill walking shrank fat cells by about 18 percent. Other studies have shown exercise is effective at reducing the deep and dangerous visceral fat that accumulates around internal organs.[276]

Dozens of studies have been conducted on the relationship between physical activity and cancer. Some findings were more encouraging than others. According to the National Cancer Institute, the strongest positive correlation relates to colon cancers, where risk reductions of 30 to 40 percent have been charted. Various studies indicated exercise can reduce the risk of breast cancer anywhere from 20 to 80 percent among pre- and postmenopausal women. High levels of moderate and vigorous physical activity during adolescence may be especially protective.

Regarding heart disease, physical activity can add one to fours years to life, largely by offsetting or delaying the effects of cardiovascular problems, according to a review of 40 years of data following more than 5,000 people in the Framingham, Mass. heart study. Exercise makes a difference not only in how long you live, but how long you enjoy a healthy life, said a researcher in the 2005 study. Another large study showed that age, fitness levels, and cardiovascular risk factors were stronger predictors of longevity than body fat.[277]

For people who already have Type 2 diabetes, exercise can help control blood sugar and keep the disease from worsening.

275: "Obese Can Improve Their Health Without Diets. Study:Lifestyle Changes Lower Risks Even Without Significant Weight Loss." *Reuters*, as posted on *MSNBC.com*. December 4, 2006.
276: "Middle-Aged Women Find It Takes More than Diet to Reduce The Abdomen." *seniorjournal.com*. August 7, 2006.
277: Rob Stein. "Exercise Can Add Nearly Four Years To Life, Study Says." *Washington Post* via *mercurynews.com*. November 15, 2005.

Even a half hour of light exercise per day is helpful to desk workers. Those who take time to get out of the office report they feel more productive and less stressed than when they don't exercise. Yoga, in particular, seems to help people with chronic low-back pain.

Think you're too old to start exercising? Volunteers in a University of South Florida study with an average age of 83 ½ years showed significant increases in body strength, flexibility and agility after participating in an exercise program of walking or resistance training for just 16 weeks. Seniors, please note the exercise was more akin to beachcombing than beach volleyball.

Are you afraid your heart's not up to it? That is something for individuals to discuss with their physicians. But a Johns Hopkins study of men and women age 55 to 75 -- all in good health but with mild, untreated hypertension -- showed that a regimen of moderate exercise improved the heart's pumping capacity without contributing to a harmful increase in heart size.[278]

THE WILLPOWER MUSCLE

Although many physicians and health professionals (especially the thinner ones) continue to urge patients to get regular exercise, there was an official turning point in 2003 when a medical advisory board to the U.S. Public Health Service simply threw in the towel. There was no longer any value in encouraging doctors to recommend exercise, the panel said, because there was no proof that patients followed such advice. One study around that time showed that follow-up telephone calls from doctors or nurses made no difference. Another study found that a year after heart surgery, only one cardiac patient in four was still exercising as prescribed.[279]

Some would consider this evidence of moral failure. Yet, it's not a complete cop-out to say our willpower muscles get too tired to work. That was the thoroughly studied and equally unsettling conclusion of researchers at Case Western Reserve University.

Psychologists Mark Muraven and Roy F. Baumeister considered several alternatives but kept coming back to the conclusion that *self-control is a limited*

278: "Message to Older Adults: Embrace, Don't Fear the Effects of Sensible Exercise." *Johns Hopkins Medical Institutions* news release. July 27, 2006.
279: Richard Lovett, Ph.D. "Refusing to Budge: Why Aren't Overweight Americans Taking Doctors' Advice to Exercise?" *Psychology Today.* January-February 2003.

resource. They reviewed other studies which involved teasing volunteers with off-limits foods, then watching them crack while attempting to solve unrelated, unsolvable puzzles. They quantified how not eating a piece of pie takes more effort than eating it. They studied how coping with stress and resisting temptation depletes self-control. And they documented how, as a direct result, subsequent efforts to manage completely unrelated temptations are less successful.

These findings can be isolated to make an attractive excuse, but take this information as a point of caution, not a season pass for self-indulgence. The same researchers showed that with repeated practice and rest, the self-control "muscle" becomes stronger over time.[280] It follows that making a habit of physical activity and sensible eating can leave your willpower muscle in better shape to deal with unusual and unexpected sources of stress. You'll be better prepared to step into fresh dog poo on your way out the door, respond to a boss gone ballistic, or maintain the will to live when your internet goes down.

MIND OVER MATTERS

The fitness message is everywhere. Public services announcements urge us to "start moving." Fitness clubs begin heavy advertising the day after Christmas. And every jogger on the street, whether clad in ostentatious red spandex or modest grey sweats, is one more reminder that others may be succeeding where you have failed.

Perhaps you're doing plenty already and just need an attitude adjustment.

Dissolve to a scene of a hotel housekeeper pushing her overloaded cart past the glass windows of the exercise room where buff road warriors are getting in their reps and tread-miles before enjoying a breakfast of melon slices and raisin bran. At least they're not the ones spilling batter all around the waffle flipper, she says to herself.

The maid has her own full day to manage. Pushing a vacuum, changing sheets, scrubbing tubs and sinks, scooting furniture back where it belongs and, when the last toilet bowl is certified fresh, walking five blocks to a bus stop and heading home where dirty laundry and dishes await.

280: Mark Muraven and Roy F. Baumeister, Case Western Reserve University. "Self-Regulation and Depletion of Limited Resources: Does Self-Control Resemble A Muscle?" *Psychological Bulletin,* 2000. Vol. 126, No. 2.

Why the gee-darn heck would she even think about paying to join a snooty fitness club? And why would I devote this much space to a vivid portrait of blue collar labor if I didn't have a really cool study to go with it?

Ta-da! Harvard psychologist Ellen Langer chose to study a group of 84 equally hard-working hotel maids. She quickly confirmed that their daily work routines alone were sufficient to exceed the U.S. surgeon general's recommendation for daily exercise. Even so, the maids' basic health measurements said otherwise.[281]

Because you're an expert on constructing scientific studies by now, you know as well as any Harvard brainiac you'd start by dividing the maids into two similar groups, then ignoring the half that will serve as the control group. Now here's the part you probably didn't think of: Langer and colleagues met with the other maids, carefully reviewing their daily work rhythms and explaining how many calories each task burned. These maids were each assured they were already engaged in a government-approved active lifestyle. That was it. No lectures, no pep talks, no brochures with happy pictures of fruits and vegetables.

A month passed. The Harvard crew returned and repeated the basic health assessment given at the start of the study. As expected, there was no change in the control group. But the maids who were given the fitness information had lost weight, improved their waist-to-hip ratio and experienced a 10 percent drop in blood pressure.

The housekeepers and their managers confirmed their work routines had not changed in any way. No veggie platters in the break room, no lunch breaks spent in the fitness room.

The psychologists believe the only change occurred between the ears of the maids in the non-control group. Activities were the same, but the simple sharing of information had triggered a mind reset. Some experts not involved in the study were skeptical, suspecting the maids had become more active away from work or were eating more healthfully. But Langer and other experts in placebo response say there is growing evidence the placebo effect is not merely subjective, but can manifest in physically measurable ways. In this case, the

---

281: Alex Spiegel. "Hotel Maids Challenge The Placebo Effect." National Public Radio, Morning Edition. *npr.org.* January 3, 2008.

maids believed they were exercising and their bodies responded accordingly.

As athletic coaches like to say, training can only take you so far.

The rest is attitude.

"Don't make an artificial distinction between exercise and physical activity," says Harvey B. Simon, M.D., another Harvard educator. A dedicated distance runner and aerobics advocate, Simon had the courage to fact-check 22 studies which showed how even moderate exercise delivers significant health benefits as measured by longevity, heart disease, diabetes, dementia, fractures, breast cancer and colon cancer.

"Intensity is great," Simon says, "but what matters most is that you simply get moving."[282]

Simon still believes that aerobics are necessary to attain maximum fitness, but his advice to real people in a real world is to not sweat the details.

Perhaps your own home could use a good housekeeping?

EXPECT LESS, GET MORE

Without dismissing the benefits of targeted or aerobic exercise, it's worthwhile to discuss some popular assumptions with your physician or trainer, who may not agree with any of the following, newer lines of thinking now making headlines.

- Crunches and sit-ups won't get rid of stomach fat. Although exercise will burn calories and eventually influence fat distribution, your body will decide where fat is stored, largely based on genetics and thereby defeating most attempts at spot reducing. Nevertheless, improving tummy muscles may improve appearances.

- Yo-yo exercising creates problems by giving your body confusing signals, just like yo-yo dieting. But it's not true that muscle cells will turn into fat cells if you abandon a regular exercise program. Yes, you

282: Harvey B. Simon, M.D. "Big Benefits From Small Changes: You Don't Have to Break a Sweat to Improve Your Health, You Just Need to Get Moving." *Newsweek* January 16, 2006. See also Simon's 2006 book, *The No Sweat Exercise Plan: Lose Weight, Get Healthy, and Live Longer.* McGraw-Hill.

may add fat, but the muscle cells will still be there -- just a little harder to find. Homeostasis stacks the deck against you. Among distance runners, we know that weight gained following a reduction in weekly foot-miles will not disappear just by returning to the previous routine.

- Stretching is good, but for most people, it's not necessary before exercising to prevent injuries. Instead, some experts say a few minutes of warm-up is more useful. Stretching can maintain flexibility after a workout, especially with weight training.

- Running doesn't ruin your joints -- if they're good to start with. Repetitive, high-impact activity can weaken an already injured knee. Healthy people can hold up well with proper technique, good shoes and a route with grassy surfaces.

- Women who train with weights won't look like men who train with weights. Anabolic testosterone in men makes it possible, but not easy, for males to bulk up, but typical strength training programs for women, including Pilates, provide benefits without the bulk.[283]

- Scratch this excuse, ladies: Sudden cardiac death during exertion is an extremely rare event among women. To the contrary, regular moderate, even vigorous, exercise may significantly lower the long-term risk.[284]

WALK THIS WAY

By all means, start moving or moving more. Researchers say obese people average sitting 2 1/2 hours a day more than their lean peers.

Beginners just need to turn off the TV, dress appropriately for the weather and get out of the house at least three times a week, for at least 10 minutes. Being able to walk 30 minutes per day, four or more days a week, doesn't take long to achieve and will have substantial fitness benefits.

Overweight people already have one advantage when walking. They burn more calories and get more value from walking slowly.

283: Joseph Brownstein. "Working Out the Kinks in 10 Exercise Myths." *ABC News Medical Unit*, February 4, 2009.
284: "Exercise Unlikely To Cause Sudden Cardiac Death in Women." *American Medical Association* news release via Newswire. March 16, 2006.

So enjoy the left-right rhythm of walking. Walk your dog. Walk your neighbor's dog. Park at the far end of the parking lot. Take the stairs at work. Take a walk during lunch breaks. Take the stairs to less-convenient bathroom at work. Walk the mall. Walk the grocery. Walk around the block and meet some neighbors. Walk with a friend and chat your socks off. Walk solo with earphones and listen to some music or an audiobook. Walk in the park or around a lake.

Walk and lose that stress. Walk and enjoy the fresh air. Walk and think about how it will leave you with a "good tired."

WORK YOUR SLEEP

That stress-reducing walk to nowhere has an important additional benefit. It improves sleep. Managing stress, sleeping well and being active each contribute to health and provide extra strength to make wiser decisions throughout the day, including the many challenging choices involving calories.

There may be a chemical connection between sleep and eating. New research suggests sleep deprivation lowers the amount of leptin, the blood protein that helps suppress appetite, while also increasing the appetite stimulant ghrelin. One study showed those hormone levels were about 15 percent out of whack for people who routinely slept just five hours per night. And you know from experience that sleep deprivation has a negative impact on memory, moods and behavior. The average adult gets 6.9 hour of sleep on weekdays, and 7.5 hours on weekends -- a daily average of seven hours. Whether or not you are getting enough sleep might best be answered by your family, friends, and coworkers. It's not hard to recognize the symptoms when the under-slept among us are less productive, unfocused, mistake-prone, grumpy and combative. If that describes you on a typical day, then it's time to review these widely agreed-upon basics of getting a good night's rest. Pay special attention to the ones you are already aware of, but have chosen to ignore.

Ready? Set. Snooze!

- Plan to sleep. Schedule to sleep. Allow time to sleep -- about seven to eight hours per night. That's how long it takes to get through three to five complete sleep cycles per night, each including a phase of conked-out, dream-inducing, brain-rebooting, rapid eye movement.

- Keep it regular, seven days a week, with a target time for lights-out and getting up. If your work hours or the solar schedule create complications, use blackout shades on windows and a "white noise" generator to block out other disturbances.

- Begin winding down hours in advance. Limit or avoid caffeine (duh), alcohol, nicotine and sugars. Don't go to bed hungry or stuffed. Know your bladder schedule and work with it.

- Do not make a habit of napping. If necessary, cat-nap in the early afternoon. Some experts say 10 to 30 minutes is plenty, and an hour is the maximum.

- Use the bedroom only for sleeping (or amusing physical activities). Make it a restful place, not an office, entertainment center, or hub for family gatherings.

- Invest in a good mattress as often as necessary, probably every five to 10 years. People keep getting bigger and beds keep getting better. This is one queen-sized slice of heaven you can't afford to scrimp on.

- Don't try to resolve personal and professional concerns with your head on a pillow. Well before bedtime, write down your to-do list or action plan for tomorrow, then leave it outside the bedroom and give your worries the night off. The problems will look a lot more manageable after a good night's rest.

- Read a good book in bed, possibly less entertaining than *Fat, Smart, Happy*. There are many which fit that category. A real book, fiction or non-fiction, will promote linear thinking, focus and relaxation -- just the opposite of the scattershot stimulation blasting from Instagram shares and tweets from twits. Save that social media upchuck for morning coffee.

- Sleep like a caveman. Keep it quiet, dark and cool enough that a blanket feels good. Crack a window, even in winter. Rely on an old-fashioned analog clock with an assertive alarm. It doesn't matter that you can't read the clock face in the dark. That's a feature! Keeping track of how long you've been awake will only add to your stress about getting back to sleep. If you're wide awake for long, get up and do something useful, albeit relaxing, until you're bored and real sleep beckons.

• Don't get stressed about sleeping. That's counter-productive, like rushing to get home before you have an accident. I've raised you to be smarter than that.

STOP STRESSING ABOUT STRESS

If you've ever turned to comfort food during times of stress, you're not alone. If you do it often, you've got some belly fat to show for it. At least that was the result for some volunteer rats in a series of University of California-San Francisco studies. The rats which were stressed out by spending more time in a confined space ate less healthy food and consumed more sugar water. Their binge therapy actually reduced measurable stress hormones, but it also added more abdominal fat. Same thing in earlier studies with stress-induced monkeys given access to an American style diet. Similarly, researchers believe the cortisol hormone which humans produce under stress causes fat stores to be relocated and deposited deep in the abdomen.

Continuous exposure to stress has also been linked to hypertension, heart disease and stroke. Stress also takes a toll on memory, problem-solving skills and the immune system. Stress could be the cause of your back pain, headache, fatigue, depression, upset stomach, constipation or diarrhea, so think about how to treat the cause, not the symptoms.

Those who are most successful at managing stress have learned proactive techniques to minimize exposure to stressful situations and to manage the ones that can't be avoided. We only add to stress by trying to control the uncontrollable. If you really don't want it to rain on your big weekend trip, pack an umbrella and boots. Save you super-powers for controlling how you *react* to life's challenges and disappointments, large and small.

Eat smart. Move more. Cut caffeine. Respect sleep time.

Minimize daily stressors. Leave early for work instead of trying to speed through traffic. Put more distance between yourself and a troublesome co-worker. Give the boss some slack -- you're probably the one stressing her out. Make a realistic to-do list that distinguishes between what is urgent and what is important, allocating the appropriate time for each. Insist that co-workers respect your time and privacy, and do the same for them. Know when to ask for help. Know when to say "No." Make some time to walk, breathe and be alone.

Put failures into perspective, then put 'em to bed. Accept that things don't always go your way. Talk it out. Replace anger with forgiveness. Turn your own mistakes into teaching moments and expect better results the next time.

If you still can't see the florist for the bees, learn some more deliberate relaxation techniques such a meditation. Or pick up some books on stress management. Or let a professional counselor help you chart a new course to happiness. You know your car runs better after an oil change and your computer perks up after clearing cookies and junk files. Give yourself the same consideration when it comes to paid, professional maintenance.

I happen to know you're worth it. Kisses, y'all!

PART THREE
READY FOR THE WORLD

22

SELF-ACCEPTANCE

RIGHTEOUS ACTIVISM FOR BEGINNERS

Doing the math on this whole self-esteem thing would be so much simpler if we could remove weight bias from the equation. I say with only a smidgen of exaggeration that the amount of self-loathing created by full-length mirrors and bathroom scales completely defies logic, justice, and humanity.

Nearly half of the 4,000 people responding to an online survey conducted by Yale University said they would give up a year of their life rather than be fat!

That's purely a hypothetical compact, I presume, unless some TV producers can find a legal way to convert the concept into a new reality show. Just for the sake of discussion, I'd want to know if this devil's bargain was tied to cancelling any year of my choice, or only the last year, which might be characterized by chemotherapy, bedpans or wandering lost in the woods in my big and tall Yoda pajamas.

The survey responses to slightly more realistic scenarios were actually the most troubling. Between 15 and 30 percent of respondents said that to be guaranteed a fat-free life they would be willing to become alcoholics, walk away from a marriage or give up the possibility of having children! Five percent would rather lose a limb than be fat! Four percent, given the option, would choose blindness!

(I do not insert exclamation marks willy-nilly. Here, I was genuinely gobsmacked.)

At least the adults who chose blindness wouldn't have to look at themselves in the mirror or give their own fat children the stink eye. Really. Ten percent of the survey group said they'd rather have a child dealing with anorexia than obesity; 8 percent thought that having a child with a learning disorder wouldn't be as bad as having a fat child.

"We were surprised by the sheer number of people who reported they would be willing to make major sacrifices to avoid being obese," said Yale's Marlene Schwartz. "It drives home the message that weight bias is powerful and pervasive."

And unhealthy. The American obsession with weight loss is not realistic or proportional. The so-called cures and collateral damage are frequently more harmful than the obesity "disease" under attack. Everyone carries a history of successes and failures, both real and imagined, modest and exaggerated.

The imperfect sum of these ups and down appears on the bottom line as self-esteem. Folks with low self-esteem have difficulty concealing it. Symptoms run the gamut of hypersensitivity, pessimism, negativity, irritability, and hostility. Some may display a crippling fear of making a mistake or an over-the-top need to please others.

There is no need to raise your hand if you see yourself in the above descriptions. If several describe you, it might explain why the last get-together you were invited to was a pity party.

ASSERTIVE COPING

But cheer up! As a card-carrying Human Being and member for life, you likely display an equal number of characteristics of high self-esteem. You have many strong values and guiding principles you love to defend. You try to learn from the past and plan for the future. You generally trust your own judgment but are not afraid to ask for help when you need it. And you are sensitive to the needs and feelings of others. Clearly you in particular and my hand-picked readers in general are an all-around fine bunch of people. Either that, or I'm just demonstrating an excessive need to please others.

We know the human body has a primal need to store fat and prepare for famine. It's once-essential survival mechanism is now grossly out of date in an era of desk jobs, an endless supply of cheap calories, and profit-minding marketing. We know that our bodies have a powerful failsafe system to prevent weight loss. And a few of us know that in any group of 100 dieters, only a handful will maintain weight loss more than two years, and that repeated weight cycling will create its own set of health problems.

And yet the widespread belief persists among fat and thin alike that being overweight or obese is a choice and therefore deserving of the hateful stereotypes that go with it. And so, fat folks engage in a variety of coping techniques, some better than others.

Some will avoid going to the mall or eating in public, rather than risk extra exposure to fatphobic ridicule. Psychologists say those who engage in self-blaming, isolation and avoidance of confrontation are more likely to experience stress and depression.

Heavy Americans who cling to the hope of shedding weight forever often side with their tormentors and willingly wear their negative stereotypes. In so doing, they'll enjoy a brief, satisfying connection with The Walking Thin. But researchers believe internalizing the biases of fat-haters only contributes to depression, hostility, binge-eating, crying, or violent outbursts.

Fortunately, research indicates that most fat people are stronger than that, and I don't just mean the ability to remove a sticky lid from a jar of marshmallow cream. Usually, coping involves a combination of more upbeat responses -- assertively heading off negative remarks in mid-sentence, positive self-talk, enjoying the support of friends, refusing to hide, turning to prayer and faith, or deploying a well-timed comeback joke.

You know where my sentiments lie, so let's go straight to an expert in the well-tempered put-down, the fabulous fat activist Marilyn Wann. Her 1998 manifesto, *Fat! So? (Because You Don't Have to Apologize for Your Size)*, remains must-reading for the fat acceptance movement. Wann and her contributors shared some choice comebacks to insults better left unsaid:

Are you pregnant? Nope. But hell, the night is young!"

How much do you weigh? A number far too large for someone with a single-digit IQ to understand.

You'd look great if you just lost some weight. Yes, but then who would you have to feel superior to?

You've put on weight! Yes! (Arms thrown wide.) My genes are expressing themselves!

Aren't those super? Isn't that what the military would call a measured and appropriate response to a deliberate attack? Don't they make you want to strut? If that gives you a whole new way of thinking about your inner self and outer fattitude, right on and read on! The Fat Majority is finding its voice.

Afraid to get on board? You probably just need a pep talk, and I know just the people to give you one. Here's some good advice from two other pioneers in the fat acceptance field -- Francie M. Berg (healthyweight.net), author of Women Afraid to Eat and similar titles, and Carol A. Johnson, author of Self-Esteem Comes in All Sizes:

- Recognize that beauty, health and strength comes in all sizes. Weight is a poor measure of self worth. See yourself as a total person -- the way you treat others, your contributions to your family, friends and community.

- Your weight is just your weight. Don't give it any more importance than that. Your body has its own opinion about how much is enough and a natural set point that can be nearly impossible to change. It's like that office building thermostat with a locked Lucite cover to keep your busy fingers out.

- Don't obsess with food being good or bad. Instead, enjoy foods that are "good to eat frequently" as well as foods that are "good to enjoy occasionally."

- Avoid "globalizing." Instead of saying "I'm such a failure," say: "I didn't do that one little thing quite right, but I do most things right."

- Don't fret about getting what you want. Want what you have. Find contentment in the abundance all around you. You also are entitled to dreams, so follow them now. Put nothing on hold as an eventual reward for out-of-reach weight loss. Just do it!

- Surround yourself with positive, supportive people. Tell friends why you have a new, weightless way to measure self-worth and tell them what the research really says about obesity. Become a role model for other adults and children by projecting confidence, self-respect and tolerance for those most in need of it.

- Fitting in does not mean caving in. Resist being passive or aggressive. Instead, just live assertively -- be open, honest and direct in expressing your feelings and opinions. You've got something worth saying (usually), so say it.

- Tight clothes may have sentimental value, but they are not comfortable or flattering. Get rid of clothes that don't fit to make room for clothes that project confidence and success. Breathing is wonderful and healthy. Choose clothes that give you room to inhale when you stop and smell the coffee.

- Remember that capitalism is behind the marketing to herd men and women toward an "ideal" image or shape. But perfection is a ruse. We don't have flaws. We have features. The human race is manufactured in an infinite variety of colors, sizes and shapes. Don't be ashamed or conceited if your shape just happens to provide more warmth in winter and shade in summer.

- Concentrate on developing a healthy lifestyle, not losing weight. Be active just for the fun of it. Normalize your life by being regularly active and keeping yourself well nourished without dieting. Balance is everything. If your doctor can't agree with the principles of health at any size, give him the sermon or shop for a doctor who gets it.

FAT CLUBS ON A MISSION

If quilters, kayakers and collectors of Monkees memorabilia can form their own clubs, you'd think there would be organizations to promote fat acceptance. Such groups have existed for 45-plus years. They were never secretive, but have only recently gained wider exposure and clout because of the same mechanism supporting new revolutions around the world -- the internet. Not surprisingly, most fat acceptance groups were created by fat women, for fat women. Men are welcome, of course, if only to set up tables and smoke a pig for a Saturday get-together. Occasional conventions provide an opportunity to socialize, swap diet horror stories, attend workshops, enjoy a flashy fat fashion show and plunge into a fat-only night at the hotel swimming pool. But the year-round importance of such organizations is to provide useful resources for members and an organized front to battle the forces of hate, discrimination, and ignorance. It's like the Rebel Alliance, if Princess Leia bore three kids and couldn't shake the weight. For those with an activist streak, challenging the status quo is where the real fun lies.

Founded in the Power-To-The-People heydaze of 1969, the Oakland, California-based National Association to Advance Fat Acceptance encompasses all the above activities and agendas. The official NAAFA to-do list for public policy-makers is political, powerful and pure. Here it is:

Employment: Include weight in the Civil Rights Act or create separate federal anti-discrimination legislation based on weight and seek inclusion in anti-discrimination policies of major corporations and institutions.

Health Care: Encourage health care organizations to adopt a Health At Every Size policy and include HAES in patients' rights policies.

Education: Protect overweight children from bullying and intimidation in school by requiring states and/or school districts to adopt HAES and enforce policies prohibiting harassment, intimidation, or bullying on school property.

NAAFA will certainly need more members to loosen a few bricks in the massive wall of fatphobic hate and fear, but NAAFA leaders such as Wann and Peggy Howell do jump at the occasional invitation from national news media to explain their far-out ideas about fairness and equality. Invariably, that begins with tamping down Misconception No. 1 -- that NAAFA is all about encouraging everyone to get fat or stay fat. Health and fitness are important and possible for everyone, they say, over and over and over. You should read about NAAFA over and over at www.naafaonline.com.

IT'S POLITICS. IT'S LOCAL.

Christianity, fantasy football, and Spanx all started with a small but dedicated cult following. And even though it may take years for Congress to even consider expanding civil rights to people of all sizes, it takes only one person or a van load of organizers to make a thoughtful presentation before a local school board, city council, or group of hospital trustees.

Think globally. Act locally. Avoid harsh demands or requests that are expensive to implement, and you'll be surprised how eager community leaders are to sign a proclamation and tweak some policies. Get resources from NAAFA, or go our own way. Grow your base by sponsoring seminars and speakers with local church, civic, and college groups. Get some other interest groups on your team, get some small successes under your belt, and build on those at the regional or state level.

Passion is helpful; facts are a must. Feel free to distribute multiple copies of this book at your own expense. Or buy yourself a nice, new outfit and download internet freebies from my website and those maintained by NAAFA and others. Check out the Yale Rudd Center for Food Policy & Obesity, The Association for Size Diversity and Health, The Council on Size & Weight Discrimination, the International Size Acceptance Association (for professionals), author Linda Bacon's HAES Community site and author Frances M. Berg's Healthy Weight Network. Some websites are useful even without frequent updates, but also look for new fat friends on Facebook and newer social networks.

Just how smart can we get? On university campuses, where it's considered hip to offer a class on "Religion and The Simpsons" or "The Grateful Dead: A Viral Marketing Case History," proponents of fat studies are still finding resistance based on the usual condemnations about weight and health. Proponents ride the elephant into the room, arguing that the societal and political consequences of obesity and discrimination deserve an airing somewhere in the humanities and social sciences. Short of creating specific courses, many professors have managed to incorporate some discussion of fat politics into established coursework on history, sociology, exercise physiology, law or women's studies.

The resistance to legitimizing fat studies echoes the entrenched reluctance of academia, not many years ago, to legitimize gender and African-American studies, even though all three are clearly connected as battlegrounds of social justice.

Traditionalists such as Stephen H. Balch, president of the conservative National Association of Scholars, have heard it all before. "In one field or another, passion and venting have come to define the nature of what academics do. Ethnic studies, women's studies, queer studies -- they're all about vindicating the grievances of some particular group. That's not what the academy should be about," he once told the New York Times. To which psychology professor Elena Escalera countered:

"This is not about victimhood, but about becoming empowered. Did Martin Luther King and Malcolm X espouse victimhood? Did Susan B. Anthony? It's really easy for people to feel that fat people are trying to find an excuse."

Phhft! The truth does not need an excuse.

HELL WELL RAISED

Sometimes it just takes a wildfire to create a volunteer fire department. Within the span of a few weeks in early 2012, a relative handful of bloggers and activists succeeded in persuading two massive organizations to back down on their ill-conceived campaigns to fight childhood obesity by clumsily shaming fat kids. In Chapter 20, "Homefront," I told you about the "Strong4Life" campaign in Georgia where a coalition of the well-intentioned but misguided created stark billboards and TV spots which only succeeded in empowering bullies with its message that fat kids are sick, lazy losers. NAAFA condemned the campaign via the few media outlets that called for a comment. More likely, the turning point was when mommy blogger Leah Segedie organized other bloggers, fanned wider resistance with Twitter events and – following the money! -- questioned the managers of a clothing store which indirectly financed the shame game. Suddenly, Strong4Life sponsors were open to a dialogue and the billboards came down.

Perhaps those billboard leases were expiring anyway, but the strong4life. com program responded with a complete makeover. The positive, multifaceted campaign now includes a school nutrition program, summer camps and a hospital-sponsored clinic.

Witness: "Created specifically for families struggling with health issues related to weight, the Strong4Life Clinic provides a warm and nurturing environment of specialized pediatric-trained team members including a Board-certified obesity medicine pediatrician, a dedicated pediatric psychologist as well as a staff of registered dietitians, exercise physiologists and other wellness experts." After this amazing 180-degree turnaround, the Strong4Life template has become one which any community would be wise to emulate. All the tools and inspiration are available at its website. Your own community may already have many of the same programs and policies in place. Find out. Reach out. Speak out.

BROCCOLI GUNS

Let's see if Mickey Mouse is smart enough to get on board. You know the Disney Empire abhors controversy the same way Donald Duck hides from speech therapists. Imagine the corporate cringing when Walt Disney World's Epcot Center came under fire immediately after unveiling a colorful, "imagineered" exhibit for kids called "Habit Heroes." Inside the attraction, sponsored by major health insurance companies, kids were educated about the dangers of spending too much time with TV and video games. Colorful costumed characters added to the adventure. The buff pair of heroes -- Will Powers and Callie Stenics – required some fat and lazy villains to bring down. Responding to a dangerous snack attack, the heroes target sugary foods with their broccoli guns. The fat and lazy villains Snacker and Lead Bottom are then forced to exercise.

This may have provided some positive reinforcement to vacationing children already in a relationship with kale and a private soccer club. But what was the takeaway message for most fat children? Just the usual: That all fat people are lazy, exercise-hating villains.

Within days after the soft opening of Habit Heroes, wire stories about Snacker and Lead Bottom grabbed the attention not only of experienced fat activists, but also parents and mainstream health professionals, all the way from Okeechobee to Ontario.

"It's so dumbfounding it's unreal," said Dr. Yoni Freedhoff, an assistant professor of family medicine at the University of Ottawa. "I just can't believe somebody out there thought it was a good idea to pick up where the school bullies left off and shame kids on their vacation."

On Monday, Feb. 27, 2012, three weeks after it opened, Disney shut down Habit Heroes and its marketing program for an indefinite "test and adjust phase." NAAFA's Peggy Howell hoped the exhibit would do away with its stigmatizing stereotypes if it reopened. She was encouraged that the Disney experiment brought needed attention to weight-based stereotyping. And it really mattered. After a 10-month lockdown, the colorful, kiddy seminar reopened, minus all the offending stereotypes, and focused on positive messages about nutrition and exercise.

NAAFA was also able to claim part of the credit in 2008 when it condemned a bill filed in the Mississippi state legislature that would prohibit the state's restaurants from serving people who are obese, with criteria to be established by the state's health department. The bill was killed in committee after a quick uproar. One sponsor of the measure later said he was merely trying to draw attention to Mississippi's highest-in-the-nation obesity rate, but he was surprised when media began calling from New York, London and Australia.

"You take food away from fat people -- my gosh," said State Rep. Ted Mayhall.

Sort of like when you take stereotypes and grandstanding away from politicians?

A month later, a hospital in Victoria, Texas came under fire for its policy to promote a more professional appearance among staff by blocking job applicants with visible tattoos and piercings -- or a body mass index above 35. After an immediate onslaught of criticism, including the suspicion the weight limits were veiled racism, the administration put the hot policy where it belonged -- in a cold bedpan.

WINNER, WINNER, CHICKEN DINNER

For individuals, there are two clear paths to choose from. The unhappy one is to continue hating yourself for year after hellish year while waiting to discover that one permanent weight-loss trick that every other self-loather somehow managed to overlook.

The happy choice begins with flipping your self-esteem switch from "Loser" to "Winner." This immediately pulls the curtain back on a heavenly world that was always there to enjoy. As a Fat, Smart and Happy woman or man, you'll enjoy the full rights and privileges required to do this:

- Eat your choice of salad or cheese fries in a public restaurant, knowing that either one is going to annoy someone who has their own hang-ups to sort out.

- Trade your judgmental "friends" for real friends who know and love the real you.

- Run your own business or climb the corporate ladder, just by doing good work and expecting respect.

- Ride a bicycle, hike in the woods, or enjoy an extra jiggly game of volleyball at a topless beach. Anything goes when you exercise because you enjoy it, not because you have to.

- Pick up a journal, a paint brush, or a musical instrument, and share your talent with a cat, the neighbors, or the whole darn world.

- Dress in a way that shows everyone you are an attractive, confident and complete person. Expect your superficial detractors to be confused or jealous of your poise. This will be their awkward phase, not yours, so make them feel just a little bit smaller, I mean better, by demonstrating patience and understanding.

- Enjoy your strength, stamina, and magnificent omnipresence. Become a masked crime-fighter, or just lend a strong hand to lesser mortals when they need help carrying a sack of dog food or case of copier paper.

- Give your tight clothes to Goodwill. Give yourself comfortable, attractive new outfits and a makeover. Draw attention to yourself -- on your terms.

- Watch as your detractors slowly forget why they used to dismiss you. Slowly convert their disrespect to admiration.

- Enjoy winter wrapped in your own cuddly insulation, along with a tall cup of cocoa.

- Watch "Hairspray" with fresh, hot popcorn while cheering for Edna and Tracy Turnblad.

I'll finish with this important reminder: Your home is not a Turkish prison. Let nary a day pass without some quality dark chocolate.

23

DISCRIMINATION NATION

Part 1 / PRIDE AND PREJUDICE

Now that you're learning to love your own fluffy self, we just need to work on the airhead attitudes of a few bajillion other people. The list of fat-haters in your life probably includes a disturbing number of folks who are supposed to be on your side: friends, teachers, classmates, your doctor, your own mother. Others, including coworkers and sassy sales clerks, remain on standby to remind you that your weight does not fit their definition of normal and healthy.

Sometimes you can expect more empathy from a total stranger. But don't count on it. Cloaked in anonymity, one reader managed to cover all the bias bases in response to a newspaper's online chat about extending discrimination laws to protect the obese:

"Is anyone else as tired of all these whiny people as I am? It used to be just women and blacks, and then the gays and transvestites. Now fat people are chiming in because they can't refrain from slamming that pair of bacon triple cheese Whoppers for breakfast every morning. Genetics my patootie. At least the women and blacks have that as an excuse, lol."

Thank you, anonymous analyst hiding in the internet shadows, for taking some of the sting away from your crude comparisons and hateful stereotypes by ending with a "laughing out loud."

Among those with the decency not to verbalize their bias, it's safe to assume many of them have bought into one or more stereotypes alleging that fat people are lazy, self-indulgent and clueless about how to lose weight.

The unspoken belief is that the overweight and obese should at least be considerate enough to somehow keep a low profile and lower their expectations in life. Why, their critics wonder, do heavyweights even pretend to be normal by running for class president, applying for a job promotion, or skipping lunch to go for a jog?

Whether they are pretending to be helpful or feel justified in their cruelty, fat-haters have a gift for giving self-esteem a kick in the gut -- the pain of which is often manifest as eating disorders, isolation, loneliness, and depression.

There are monetary damages as well. Discrimination based purely on weight often means being discouraged from attending college, being denied a scholarship or bank loan, or, just to keep jolliness in check, being overlooked for a job opening or a promotion.

WEIGHT BIAS BATTLEGROUND

Weight bias is deserving to be the next civil rights battleground for the United States. The fight unfolds in a lawless frontier where even the liberal media are part of a system that not only tolerates but also promotes widespread social injustice for big people.

So you think losing 50 pounds is hard? Turning around a culture this pervasive is going to be like putting shredded cabbage back together again. One would think that today -- when two-thirds of Americans are considered overweight or obese -- fatism would be going out of style.

But no. The un-evolved messages from Hollywood, advertising agencies, fashion police, and the $55 billion dollar diet industry have managed to reinforce and expand negative weight stereotypes within a larger, fatter population.

According to a large, multi-topic survey conducted in the mid-90s and again in the mid-2000s, perceived discrimination based on race decreased during that span. Kudos, America. That's some progress.

But the prevalence of discrimination increased in four other categories:

age, gender, ethnicity, and height or weight. Reports of overt occurrences of size-based discrimination jumped to 12 percent from 7 percent during the study interval.

Because we are not hearing anything about the free world's "Shortness Epidemic," we can assume most, if not all, of the size-based prejudice reported in the survey was a matter of width or weight. In fact, discrimination increased with an individual's weight. Among the moderately obese, the incidence rate was 14.2 percent; among the severely obese, 42.5 percent. Race, age and gender were aggravating factors. For anyone other than Aretha Franklin, being fat *and* black *and* female is evidently the hardest way to gain R.E.S.P.E.C.T.. But for whatever reason, society is more forgiving as we age. Survey respondents aged 55-64 were half as likely to report size discrimination than those aged 35-44.[285] In the eye of the beholder, it seems that a sprinkle of wrinkles makes old fat more cuddly.

HEAD START ON HATE

Weight-based bias and self-loathing starts as early as age 3. Studies have documented several unsettling facts. Children are more repulsed by an obese child than by a child who was disfigured by an accident. Children buy into all the mean, ugly and stupid stereotyping. For young girls, even average weight is considered unacceptable. Among children, weight bias is more common and damaging than race discrimination. Social relationships suffer because of weight teasing, especially for girls.

Weight-based teasing and bullying in schools is so common it goes unchallenged. Even teachers, staff and parents with a more sensitive approach often contribute to the lower self-esteem of heavy children by attempting to send a positive message about dieting. Teenagers who are still not mature enough to see the value of moderation in anything may interpret dieting advice as a justification for taking diet pills, abusing laxatives, skipping meals or launching a new cycle of binge eating and purging.

285: Tatiana Adreyeva, Rebecca M. Puhl and Kelly D. Brownell. "Changes in Perceived Weight Discrimination Among Americans, 1995-1996 Through 2004-2006." *www.obesityjounral.org*. Feb. 28, 2008. The comparison was based on the National Survey of Midlife Development in the United States.

BLAME GAMES

But why the overall increase in weight bias? The analysis by the Rudd Center for Food Policy and Obesity at Yale University, which funded the research, concluded it was largely attributable to the fattening of America and the blame game surrounding it. Media buzz about obesity increased fivefold during one 11-year span, and most of that attention framed the obesity "epidemic" in terms of personal responsibility and individual solutions.

It is still very rare for obesity to be presented as the complex physiological, environmental, and societal issue it is. Hey, it was news to me, and I've been a news professional since Richard Nixon was president. Regardless, what chance would the occasional fair-and-balanced news report have in shaping public opinion?

The fat-is-ugly message is delivered non-stop by the entertainment industry and with paid television and magazine advertisements for weight loss products and techniques, all delivered with **loud, bold claims** and rapid-fire, fine-print disclosures. The weight-loss industry has a vested interest in promoting solutions which rarely achieve long-term success. Our "personal failure" to lose weight is what keeps them in business. Fatism sells zero-calorie soft drinks and diet pills and liposuction the same way racism sells suburban homes, guns and burglar alarms. It's a newer, sanitized, and profitized version of the same same old politics of fear and hate.

It's not all meanness. It's human nature to excuse your own weight gain until you are able to quit that second job, quit eating in the car, spend more time at the gym, and start cooking healthier. Our obstacles to quick weight loss are just a fact of life, we think, while everyone else facing the same challenges just lacks self-control.

At work, casual fatism is permitted, even expected. You probably wouldn't joke aloud with colleagues about another co-worker's bald spot, crooked teeth or thrift shop clothing. But if Alice in accounting doesn't snap back to the dress size she wore before birthing twins, the situation requires a robust discussion by the usual creeps and gossip-mongers.

It's not all greed and profiteering. I want to believe that the great majority of educators, policy-makers, medical professionals, and health journalists have the plus-sized public's welfare at heart. However, as vessels of Conventional Wisdom, they are inclined to emphasize long standing (and often disproved) assumptions about health and weight.

Some experts think the increased hostility toward the overweight reflects fear and self-loathing. People who are struggling with their own weight or self-esteem may transform their frustrations into anger directed toward others. This matches up with studies showing that young women are most likely to be critical of themselves because of weight -- and also exhibit the most weight bias toward others.

"There's a widespread belief that fat is controllable," says Linda Bacon, author of *Health at Every Size: The Surprising Truth About Your Weight*. She writes that with such beliefs, compassion has no place. "Now you can blame the individual and attribute all kinds of mean qualities to them."[286]

It doesn't help that obesity is usually diagnosed from across the room. No calipers, scales or blood tests are needed to confirm the appearance of multiple chins or rubbing thighs. Nor do the visual clues come with any history or explanation.

Is that fat person who is taking up more than one seat on the bus on a first-name basis with the whole crew at the doughnut shop? Or is he a former distance runner whose metabolism never adjusted to an injury and long rehabilitation? Or a vegan yoga instructor whose prescription medicine for controlling seizures, depression or high blood pressure also promotes weight gain?

In just the last few days, it is possible you had a brief encounter with a compulsive liar, a tax cheat, an arsonist, a philanderer, a spouse abuser or a child molester. There are creeps among us, but what would make you suspicious of any one in particular? Nothing would. They all get the assumption of innocence, the benefit of a doubt. Contrast that to common assumptions made about large people whose size alone is regarded as all there is to know.

MALPRACTICE BY BIAS

The overweight among us are repeatedly told their health is adversely impacted by extra pounds, yet efforts to get appropriate diagnosis and treatment

---

286: Bacon as quoted by Kate Dailey and Abby Elin. "The Fat Wars: America's Weight Rage / War on the Overweight." *www.newsweek.com.* August 26, 2009.

from medical professionals are often met with the same stigma, blame, and hostility faced in any other public place.[287] The frustrating experience leads overweight patients to delay seeking urgent care or to schedule routine visits for checkups, flu shots, mammograms, and Pap smears. Such delays only aggravate the cost and effectiveness of treatment.

More than half of overweight patients surveyed reported hearing inappropriate comments about their weight from doctors, as well as negative stereotyping from nurses, dietitians and mental health professionals. It's not just paranoia. Other studies conducted within the medical community have confirmed the same biases -- whether explicit or unspoken. Physicians are more likely to regard obese patients as awkward, unattractive, weak-willed, ugly, and noncompliant. They will assume the heavy patient is inactive and food-addicted. Usually, they will be wrong. Once in awhile they may be right in their assumptions, either by accident or by asking enough non-judgmental questions to reach the truth.

Tellingly, one survey of general practitioners in France showed those with negative attitudes toward the obese were less likely to subscribe to medical journals. Sadly, they may be less informed about new research into the complex nature of obesity than are you, my favorite open-minded and curious reader.

To be fair, physicians often feel just as confused and hopeless as their patients. Additional studies have shown they often feel poorly trained or ineffective in addressing obesity. They've learned it's easy to say the wrong thing to patients. They are afraid to be confrontational unless there is some clear evidence of hypertension or impending diabetes. It's an uncomfortable and unsatisfying part of the job. And if the physician is also overweight, then who wants to hear his advice, no matter how reasoned?

And so, the long-dreaded medical office visit -- with its stuffy waiting room and tight chairs, an embarrassing hallway climb onto weight scales, and flimsy examination table -- is cut mercifully short. The episode ends without any progress. There is just more unhealthy stress for the patient.

The people who have studied weight bias in medical settings have already

---

287: Rebecca M. Puhl and Chelsea A. Heuer. Rudd Center for Food Policy & Obesity, Yale University. "The Stigma of Obesity: A Review and Update." www.obesityjournal.org. January 22, 2009.

thought about some workable solutions, all of them corresponding with the overall need to accommodate fat people and educate the non-fat. The best procedures are simply examples of the respect and consideration any service provider should want for his customers. But here are the hallmarks of any fat-friendly medical setting.[288, 289]

- A staff that is friendly, welcoming, and positive in all dealings with all patients.

- The intention to adequately treat any patient, regardless of size. An attitude of commitment starts with sturdy, wide chairs in the waiting room, discrete weigh-ins, and generously sized supplies and equipment such as gowns, blood pressure cuffs, and examination tables.

- Physicians who demonstrate their understanding of the complex physiological and environmental contributors to obesity and maintain an empathetic, nonjudgmental attitude. Brushing up on their knowledge of behavioral theory will help physicians create a long-term partnership with patients in an atmosphere that promotes self-confidence and motivation.

- Heightened sensitivity. "Obese" may be a medically correct term, but it's a long way from becoming emotionally neutral in common usage. And "grossly obese" is never going to sound objective or considerate. The physician or the patient can help frame the weight discussion positively by focusing on strength, stamina and health. Future weigh-ins are required, but merely to provide some context. Instead, goals should address eating and exercise habits. The most meaningful results can be measured by blood pressure, simple lab reports and patient confidence.

Part 2 / WORKPLACE AND THE PRICE OF BIAS

The path to lower earnings starts after high school. Obese girls and boys

---

288: James L. Early and Judy A. Johnson. "Improving Medical Practice." Chapter 16 of *Weight Bias: Nature, Consequences, and Remedies.* Edited by Kelly D. Brownell and others. *The Guilford Press.* New York. 2005.

289: Lorraine Steefel, RN, MSN. "Nurse: Healthcare Providers Need to Lose the Blame and Hostility, and Care for the Obese." *Nursing Spectrum.* March 8, 2004.

are less likely to be accepted to the best colleges, regardless of academic ability, and once enrolled, heavier females receive less financial support from their parents. Yep, their own parents. [290]

Back in the 70s, I got to know the owner of a high-end audio shop. It was fun to stop by on my way home from work to talk music and lust over the walnut speaker cabinets, powerful stereo amplifiers, gimmicky high-end cassette recorders, and, usually, the young lady behind the front counter. The face would change once or twice a year, but the new hire would be equally attractive.

Why is it that only the best-looking young girls applied to work in a geeky stereo store, I naively asked the owner. They were not the only ones to apply, he assured me. Anyone who answered the advertisement was invited to fill out a one-page application. But before the applicants were out the door, the proprietor had penciled in a few symbols, known only to him, that made it easy to call back only the most attractive candidates for a second interview.

Today, 45 years later, men are still sexist pigs, and good-looking women still have a marketable advantage in landing a date, a husband, or a high-visibility job. But an equally common form of discrimination in hiring and employment today is easily measured by height and weight. Large people -- especially women -- have a harder time finding work and, once hired, are paid less for the privilege of working in a thin-centric world.

Study after study has proved experimentally and anecdotally that fat people are less likely to be hired, are perceived to have character traits that will negatively affect job performance, are more harshly disciplined on the job, and are paid less than their non-fat counterparts. As health insurance costs skyrocket, employers are being more open about not hiring workers perceived to be less healthy and more costly to employ. And why wouldn't employers choose to discriminate? The laws and the judges are almost always on their side.

Various studies have proved weight bias in hiring. One method was as simple as presenting employment screeners with skewed resumes. The applicants' skill set, age, and personal interests were kept constant. Only the

---

290: Janet D. Latner and Marlene B. Schwartz. "Weight Bias in a Child's World," Chapter 4 of *Weight Bias: Nature, Consequences, and Remedies*. Edited by Kelly D. Brownell and others. The Guilford Press. New York. 2005.

height and weight description of the applicants were spread over a range. The predictable result was that all the skills and interests of the heavy applicants somehow became less suitable for the job.

Other studies have been more theatrical. In a Hollywood-style study conducted at Chicago Medical School in the mid-1990s, male and female actors went through mock employment interviews which were videotaped, then repeated with elaborate make-up and prosthetics to make them appear 20 percent overweight. Then 320 male and female volunteers rated the candidates based on their printed resumes and video appearance. You can guess the overall outcome.

Also noteworthy in this study: weight bias was more pronounced among female decision-makers, especially those who were most satisfied with their own weight. The adult workplace, evidently, is just like high school where obese girls are three times more likely to be bullied than their slimmer peers. Instead of an environment where maturity and fairness have outgrown cliques and stereotypes, the modern American workplace is still a domain where females are more likely than males to be the victims *and* perpetrators of weight bias.

A trio of large studies sought to quantify weight bias in dollars and cents. After controlling for other variables including health limitations, one study figured the wage penalty for obese men ranged from 0.7 to 3.4 percent and for women, 2.3 to 6.1 percent. Another study found that for white females, being 64 pounds above "average" weight came with a wage penalty of 9 percent -- equivalent to subtracting a year and half of education or three years of work experience. Read that again. Memorize it. Share it.

A third study concluded that among white women, the weight penalty in wages ranged from 5.8 percent for the mildly obese to 24 percent for the severely obese. For black women, the fat tax ranged from 3.3 percent to 14.6 percent. Very obese white men also faced a stiff weight penalty of 19.6 percent, while the discount for the fattest black males was only 3.5 percent.[291]

Men and women of average or below weight also experience an irrational difference in favoritism as measured by compensation. Very thin men are

---

291: Puhl and Heuer, Footnote 3, above. The studies they cited were conducted by C.L. Baum and W.F. Ford (2004), J. Crawley (2004), and C.L. Maranto and A.F. Stenoien (2000).

assessed a skinny tax, then rewarded for any weight gain up the point of obesity. "For American men, gaining 25 pounds produces a predicted increase in wages of roughly $8,437 per year at below average weights, and a predicted increase of approximately $7,775 per year at above average weights." This from a pair of studies of thousands of workers in Germany and the U.S. reported in 2010.[292]

Conversely, women who satisfy the societal ideal of thinness are routinely paid more than a co-worker of average weight. But it's a short honeymoon. Those who dare to reach an average weight are deemed to have already fallen from grace and begin the penalty phase of their earnings power. Similar findings in both Germany and the U.S. "show that once women reach an average weight, subsequent weight gains are actually penalized to a lesser extent, presumably because the social preferences for a feminine body *have already been violated*," the researchers concluded.

Jeez Louise. And lawmakers would rather shake their fists and click their dentures debating who can use which public bathroom instead of addressing years of widespread, institutionalized wage discrimination based on gender and race.

THE COST TO EMPLOYERS

Employers also have a history of paying a little extra to taller employees or deducting for a foreign accent -- two variables assumed to make a difference in first impressions during the hiring process, and subsequently, with customers. But the weight issue has taken on a more calculated , long-term significance. There is a growing body of research that says fat workers miss more work, are less productive when they are on the job, and contribute to higher medical costs for their employers and co-workers.

I haven't found the research results to be entirely consistent or always pointing to the same conclusion, but for now it matters little what you or I think. Employers and their consultants are seeing the research and it validates their assumptions and stereotypes. Fat employees, in real dollars, are increasingly seen as a real liability. The rap sheet includes the cost of treating chronic ailments,

---

292: Timothy A. Judge (University of Florida) and Daniel M. Cable (London Business School). "When It Comes to Pay, Do the Thin Win? The Effect of Weight on Pay for Men and Women." *Journal of Applied Psychology.* August 20, 2010.

especially diabetes and heart disease (which have been *associated* with obesity but not consistently as a cause), as well as lost productivity resulting from injury, illness, and death. I am willing to concede that disabled or dead employees will miss their monthly sales targets.

One broad study said the percentage of medical spending in the U.S. attributable to obesity has increased steadily since at least 1998, with the biggest uptick pegged to the 2006 addition of a prescription drug benefit to Medicare. Here, a team of health economists determined the adult per capita spending attributable to obesity (inflation-adjusted here to 2017 dollars) was $1,059 in 1998, or 37 percent more than for "normal weight" people. By 2006, they say, the obesity surcharge was 41.5 percent, or $1,627. Breaking the costs down further according to type of insurance, the study showed private carriers took the biggest hit with a 58 percent obesity surcharge, versus 46.7 percent for Medicaid and 36.4 percent for Medicare.[293]

Separately, a Duke University Medical Center study showed its heaviest employees filed twice as many workers' compensation claims and missed 13 times as many work days, compared to preferred weight employees. The study covered more than 11,000 employees of Duke's health system, in and of itself a broad representation by age, gender, race and profession. Tracking their weight and medical claims over three years, the data showed employees in the "normal" BMI range filed workers' compensation claims at a rate of 5.8 per 100 full-time workers, compared to 8.81 claims for moderately obese employees and 11.65 claims among the very obese. The range in lost work days was equally disparate. [294]

One aging specialist who reviewed the Duke study conceded that obesity is a strong risk factor for many chronic conditions including osteoarthritis, diabetes and heart disease. Still, the presence of those diseases "does not explain the relationship between obesity and disability," Luigi Ferrucci, M.D. of the National Institute on Aging, said in an editorial accompanying the published study. The study's authors also noted limitations of their research. "For example, if obese nurses (because of discrimination or some other reason) are less likely to get promoted, they may be (literally) doing more of the heavy lifting." [295]

293: Eric A. Finkelstein et al. "Annual Medical Spending Attributable to Obesity: Payer and Service-Spe-
cific Estimates." *Health Affairs*. No. 5. (2009).
294: Truls Ostbye, M.D., Ph.D. and others. "Obesity and Workers Compensation." Archives of Internal
Medicine, 2007.
295: Jeff Minerd. "Obese Employees Weigh Heavily on Bottom Line." *medpagetoday.com*. April 24,

John Cawley, an expert on obesity and economics at Cornell University, also weighed in. The BMI scale used in the study didn't distinguish muscle from fat, he said, and blacks (comprising 27 percent of the Duke study group) are particularly likely to be misclassified as obese by a BMI chart obese.[296]

(Somewhat ironically, there is a huge amount of heavy lifting required in hospitals and rest homes today in the form of simply lifting obese patients in or out of chairs and beds. Walk the hallways of any nursing home. You'll see several hydraulic sling lifts lined up along the walls or already in use to make the weightiest moves possible for one or two attendants.)

HERE'S 1.7 SECONDS. GO BE MORE PRODUCTIVE.

A more recent study sought to blame overweight and obesity for 450 million additional lost work days each year. The Gallup-Healthways Well-Being Index was based on data collected in a survey of nearly 110,000 full-time employees. But what I found noteworthy was the breakdown that showed how little obesity affected productivity, even though 66 percent of workers are considered overweight or obese. Instead of only counting days missed from work, employees were asked how often "poor health" kept them from doing their "usual activities" during the previous 30 days. The results were estimated to be about three times the number of actual sick days taken.[297]

OK. The findings!

Among respondents with no health issues, the subset of overweight or obese workers reported having .36 unhealthy days per month, compared to .34 days for "normal" weight employees. That's a difference of 9 minutes, 36 second per month, or 1.7 seconds per work day.

Overweight or obese employees with three or more chronic conditions reported an average 3.51 unhealthy days per month. For "normal" weight people also coping with three or more chronic illnesses, the corresponding figure was 3.48 days per month.

2007.

296: Carla K. Johnson, Associated Press Writer. "Study: Fat Workers Cost Employers More." www.physorg.com. April 24, 2007.

297: Chronic health conditions, as defined in the study, included being overweight or obese, and/or a history of heart attack, high blood pressure, high cholesterol, cancer, diabetes, asthma, depression or chronic pain in the neck, back, knee or leg.

That's it. The heaviest, least healthy workers reported feeling unhealthy an additional 14 minutes and 24 seconds per month. The spread was the same for the category with one or two chronic illnesses: 1.08 unhealthy days per month for the overweight and obese, versus 1.07 for lightweights.[298]

Here was another stab at attaching a price to obesity. A team of number-crunchers representing the Society of Actuaries (Actual, official slogan: "Risk is Opportunity.") reviewed dozens of studies, applied dozens of calculations and concluded that in 2009 the total annual economic cost of overweight and obesity in the United States and Canada caused by medical costs, disability and "excess mortality" was about $300 billion total for the two nations.

The study gave appropriate weight, IMHO, to the science linking obesity with diabetes and cardiovascular disease -- two big drivers of costly medical treatment.

I was pleasantly surprised when these statisticians for the insurance industry broke with Conventional Wisdom right there on page 7 of their 78-page report: "Not all of the studies we reviewed reported negative effects for obesity. In fact, most research suggests that, while severe obesity *and underweight* significantly increase all-cause mortality, overweight does not appear to be a similar risk factor."[299]

HEALTH INSURANCE AND ARBITRARY PENALTIES

Wage penalties for overweight and obese employees are a common business practice. Penalties are covertly calculated and intended to offset higher medical insurance costs, according to an ongoing study for the National Bureau of Economic Research. It found that for workers in jobs *without* employer-provided health insurance, there is only a small obesity wage penalty. Predictably, the wage penalty is highest in jobs where health insurance is offered.

Because premiums in a group insurance plan are rarely adjusted for individual employee risks, employers and lower-weight employees could argue that an unofficial or "coincidental" wage offset for heavy co-workers is

---

298: Dan Witters and Sangeeta Agrawal. "Unhealthy U.S. Workers' Absenteeism Costs $153 Billion." October 17, 2011. Gallup-Healthways Well-Being Index. *www.gallup.com.*

299: Donald F. Behan, Ph.D., FSA and Samuel H. Cox, Ph.D, FSA. "Obesity and its Relation to Mortality and Morbidity Costs." *Society of Actuaries.* 2010.

a fair redistribution of costs. But the bias behind wage penalties tends to be arbitrary, unlike the hard data that goes into setting insurance premiums. As a result, research by the National Bureau of Economic Research suggests that for both male and female obese workers, *the amount of the wage penalty exceeds the expected marginal cost of providing their health benefits.*[300]

If we were more open about the process, we might find fair ways to adjust individual premiums within a group insurance plan according to weight, smoking, and all other risk factors. But so far, we're only seeing institutionalized discrimination in the form of lower wages and skipped-over promotions, based primarily and subjectively on obesity bias.

CARROTS AND CLUBS

Can we all agree that health care costs are out of control and that drug and alcohol abuse, smoking, inactivity and unhealthy eating patterns have all undermined dramatic advances in medical care? These are enormous issues made even more complicated by the posturing of regulators and the regulated, and by the inability of Congress to agree on anything other than taking another vacation and pay raise.

The reality is that most Americans get their health insurance through employers which are struggling to maintain benefits and passing a larger share of costs to the workers. Now and into the foreseeable future, employers have a vested interest in promoting wellness and reducing injuries for all employees, and not just the ones caught in the act of working while fat.

The largest, most progressive companies have been on this track for some time. One survey showed about two-thirds of employers offer on-site fitness programs and a fitness center. At the same time, two-thirds of employers also reported that only one in four workers took advantage of their fitness programs.

Give many companies credit for introducing healthier foods to cafeterias and vending machines, eliminating nearby parking and deliberately slowing down elevators while making stairwells more attractive with improved lighting,

---

300: "Why Obesity Lowers Wages." National Bureau of Economic Research. January 18, 2010. *www. nber.org.* The research cited is "The Incidence of the Healthcare Costs of Obesity," NBER Working Paper No. 11303, by Jay Bhattacharya and M. Kate Bundorf.

art, and piped-in music.

Congratulations if your employer is your best friend and deeply concerned about your personal health and well-being. The rest of us can assume the overarching goal among employers is to raise productivity and lower health costs. Not surprisingly, more companies are testing legal and ethical boundaries by trying either cash incentives or financial penalties to promote healthy habits, not just on the job, but around the clock.

In what may be a precursor to the battle against obesity, employers have already taken aim at smokers. The carrot-and-stick approach includes cash bonuses to workers who quit smoking and stay quit. Other companies prefer a club. They are adding a smoking surcharge to insurance premiums for smokers, or -- in the 20 or so states where it is legal -- even firing smokers who don't make their deadline for quitting. Needless to say, other smokers need not apply for those openings.

Some advocates for worker rights say employers are entering a slippery slope with incentives or penalties for smoking or weight loss. What gives them the right, the argument goes, to police around-the-clock personal behaviors that may have no real bearing on job performance? But, realistically -- in an era where adults willingly publicize their bad habits on Facebook, submit to drug testing and accept 24/7 on-call status as as a condition for employment -- I don't see any meaningful opposition that could reverse the trend.

Efforts to profitize wellness certainly deserve further study, especially in light of two darkly perverse ironies hiding in the shadows. According to a 2009 study funded by the Centers for Disease Control, the employer's cost of providing work site wellness programs is often greater than the cost savings from improved health. The CDC simulation estimated an annual savings of just $90 to $160 for each overweight or obese employee who sustains a 5 percent weight loss.[301] And here is a significant long-term consideration. Because of differences in life expectancy, the lifetime health expenditures are highest for people with the *best* health habits, and lowest for smokers, according to a 2008 study among the Dutch. Obese individuals fall in the middle in terms of life expectancy and

---

301: "Workplace Obesity Interventions Must Be Inexpensive to Generate a Return on Investment." RTI International. August 21, 2009. *www.newswise.com*.

health costs.[302]

Have employers and politicians just decided that fat workers are a safe scapegoat for higher health costs and lower productivity? Science writer and columnist Daniel Engber, rankled by the hyperinflation of obesity cost figures floated in the 2008 presidential campaign, said then it was time to weigh the sticker shock of obesity against "a plague of ridiculous productivity-cost estimates."

"If we believe that extra pounds result in $40 billion of lost business, what are we to make of the claim that negativity in the workplaces costs a whopping $350 billion? Spam e-mails eat away another $20 billion, and even the NCAA college basketball tournament costs us $3.8 billion. With all these other numbers floating around," Engber argued, "the cost of obesity loses all meaning."[303]

IS WEIGHT DISCRIMINATION EVEN LEGAL?

If only weight-based discrimination was a seasonal disorder, like March Madness. Instead, the bias exists year-round, virtually unchecked by national, state or local law.

While lawmakers and the courts have seen an explosion of interest in prohibiting or reversing discrimination based on race or gender, the broad rights of employers to hire and fire at will has largely sufficed to quash legal challenges based on weight bias. Often, the only viable avenue available to a victim of discrimination is to accept the knotty premise that obesity is a handicap, and therefore a protected status.

Thus far, only union-friendly Michigan and a few liberal enclaves such as Washington, D.C. and Santa Cruz and San Francisco in California have enacted laws specifically outlawing discrimination based on weight and height. Mountains of federal law bulldozed into place over the past half century have leveled the playing field for most Americans seeking fair access to work and accommodations. For obese workers, it is still a muddy, uphill slog.

302: Pieter H.M. van Baal, and others. "Lifetime Medical Costs of Obesity: Prevention No Cure for Increasing Health Expenditure." www.PLoSmedicine.org. February 2008.
303: Daniel Engber. "Abolish the Fat Tax! It's Time to Shut Up About 'The Cost of Obesity.'" *www.slate.com*. February 14, 2008.

The Civil Rights Act of 1964 ably dealt with discrimination based on gender, race, religion or national origin, but has been useful only in weight discrimination cases where weight standards were applied differently to protected classes. A 1973 law prohibited discrimination against otherwise-qualified individuals with handicaps in any program drawing federal dollars. The Americans with Disabilities Act of 1990 (ADA) boldly extended those protections to the private sector.

Since then, a handful of cases have left a patchwork of verdicts and conflicting interpretations as to whether or when obesity is an actual disability, a protected status or just an eyesore for some employers. [304] [305]

Some employers will choose hardcore resistance. "Such marketplace-driven discrimination is clearly within the rights of private sector employers," insists Patrick Basham with the libertarian Cato Institute. "If the nation's public health mandate is to produce a significantly lower level of obesity in the near term, the use of discrimination by employers is a perfectly logical and defensible instrument to employ in the war on fat." [306]

Whoa! Time out. That same free-market spirit of rejecting oversight is also used to defend the powerful corporations and trade associations that defend their undeclared war on Americans' health! They came armed with sugar-enriched foods and relentless marketing under the camouflage of creating convenient new choices for consumers.

Are the libertarians really joining a war on obesity?

Or merely trying to justify a war on fat people?

HOLLYWOOD'S REALITY NO-SHOW

Hollywood has a long history of being slightly ahead of the social justice curve with an inclusive agenda for race and gender politics. In the early 1960s, the typical Western was still depicting "redskins" and "injuns" as savage cutthroats. It took the post-Woodstock revolution to recast Native Americans

---

304: Rebecca Puhl and Kelly D. Brownell. "Bias, Discrimination and Obesity." *Obesity Research*, Vol. 9, No. 12, December 2001.
305: "Weight Discrimination Laws, Rulings, Attorneys.." *The Council on Size & Weight Discrimination*. *www.cswd.org.* Undated.
306: "Room for Debate: Should Legislation Protect the Obese?" The New York Times. *www.nytimes. com.* November 28, 2011.

as guardians of nature and survivors of the white man's genocide.

African Americans went through the same on-screen evolution, first appearing as sidekicks and servants who "happen to be black," then as black doctors and lawyers mentoring other blacks who happen to be pimps and drug-dealers.

Today, the casting of blacks shows a relaxed complacency and a new kind of stereotyping: Instead of playing a maid or a field hand, the one black face in an all-white drama is usually the tough-as-nails judge or tougher-than-nails police chief, either of which is more likely to be a woman in order to lazily fill two minority slots. Next -- hastened by the proliferation of new cable and satellite channels eager to be noticed -- Hollywood's depictions of biracial or homosexual relationships quickly went from cutting edge to cliche.

But where in TV land are the people who really look like two-thirds of Americans -- the overweight and obese men, women and children of all colors? To find the truth, we have to go to the absurdist humor of NBC's "30 Rock."

On the sketch show-within-a-sitcom, one of the characters played by the blonde narcissist, Jenna Maroney, is "Pam, the Overly-Confident Morbidly Obese Woman." At the beginning of Season 2, Jenna returns to work (in a fat suit), explaining she had put on weight starring in a summer stage adaptation of "Mystic Pizza" that required her to eat 32 slices of pizza per week. Unamused, network executive Jack Donaghy tells Jenna's supervisor, Liz Lemon: "She needs to lose 30 pounds or gain 60. Anything in between has no place in television."

And that's pretty much the way it's been in Hollywood, going back to when studio moguls were fretting about Judy Garland or Elizabeth Taylor putting on a few pounds. Today's slender starlets and buff men are paid very well to comply with the industry's fixation on fitness. The real cost is measured by the damage to the national psyche.

The millions of men, women and children watching at home -- most of them 5, 10 or 15 BMI points heavier than the stars on TV, routinely see this: Thin characters with desirable attributes dominating the central roles; overweight characters filling in the minor, stereotyped roles; thin people involved in romantic relationships; fat people lonely and losing out, preoccupied with eating and generally being ridiculed, all with the reinforcement of audience titters or a pre-recorded laugh track. This has all been quantified by studies.[307]

Fat adults accept most of this as truth and normalcy, having been subjected to a daily doses of Hollywood's fat bias as children. One study of 4,000 cartoon characters screened from 1930 to the mid-1990s showed a gradual decline of overweight characters who were shown in an unbiased light, replaced with more frequent depictions of the overweight being unattractive and unintelligent. Similarly, a more recent analysis of the most popular videos and books among children 4 to 8 portrayed thin female characters as kind, likeable and successful while heavy children played the mean and unattractive heavies in the stories.

The same imbalance carries over to TV commercials, where thin people have nothing but fun, drive new cars and enjoy frequent sex with handsome strangers while fat people are only seen in the "before" pictures for weight loss products, or as the dopey friend who drinks the wrong brand of beer.

Hollywood, never averse to making money, has made a few attempts to appeal directly to heavyweights. Before striking Oscar gold as the meanest of heavies in the film "Precious," actress-comedienne Mo'Nique promoted fat acceptance with a series of televised *Fat Chance* beauty contests for plus-sized ladies and in the film *Phat Girlz*.

Cable's Lifetime channel dealt nervously with weight issues in its fantasy courtroom dramedy *Drop Dead Diva*. Here, a thin, underachieving model dies in a car crash and returns to life in the body of a successful, plus-sized lawyer. Hilarity and heartbreak ensue as she enjoys a second doughnut and waits for her former boyfriend to recognize her inner beauty. *Diva* completed six seasons with its premise of a woman who undeservedly woke up fat one day, but at least managed to put one or two weight stereotypes under cross-examination each week.

Today, a smattering of plus-sized people have been allowed on prime-time television, including some who are confident, successful, and able to make an occasional fat joke at their own expense.

The largest and most-recognized character is Kate Pearson, one of three mismatched siblings on NBC's lovable tear-fest, *This Is Us*. Actress Chrissy

---

307: Rebecca Puhl and Kelly D. Brownell. "Bias, Discrimination and Obesity." *Obesity Research*, Vol. 9, No. 12, December 2001

Metz, who plays Pearson, knows everything about Hollywood's unwritten caste and casting system. Her "overnight" stardom followed a disheartening stretch averaging only one audition per year. Her first big role was a five-episode run in *American Horror Story: Freak Show*, playing -- what else? -- The Fat Lady.

In interviews, Metz talks about her long history of failed diets and her delicate truce with Hollywood stereotyping. "Size doesn't equate to beauty," she told the fashion magazine Marie Claire. "I don't understand why that's a thing. Well, I do, because the media has told us thin is beautiful."[308]

Even if Metz is comfortable with her own body, writers of the family melodrama are the voice of Kate Pearson: one more woman frowning at the bathroom scale, weighing the risks of weight-loss surgery or stealing away to a fat farm.

Completeness requires that I mention television's most popular and damaging fat-centric series, "The Biggest Loser." Here's a program that not only perpetuated the stereotype of self-loathing losers, but offered a dangerous blueprint for losing weight quickly. It's simple, really. Just quit your day job, sign waivers to indemnify the show's producers from medical liability, submit to filmed sessions with a drill sergeant for motivation, diet relentlessly, compete for a huge cash prize and have millions of witnesses. Off-camera, contestants were preparing for their weekly weigh-ins by fasting and exercising for hours in heavy clothing, sometimes dehydrating to the point, as one winner disclosed, of urinating blood.

The show was only recently cancelled. So, what are the chances the producers will follow up with a new series to report on each contestant's rebound weight since leaving the show? They could call it "The Biggest Gainer."

308: Marisa Meltzer. "'This Is Us' Star Chrissy Metz Takes On the F Word." March 6, 2017. *Marieclaire. com.*

24

fUN fACTORS

Thus far we've reviewed and evaluated dozens of studies. Let's conduct our own, right here, right now. Are these jokes funny? If so, which one of the two is funnier?

- You're so fat, when you sit down, the record skips -- at the radio station!

- I'm so fat, I can't even fit into a chat room!

Hmmm. Both qualify as fat jokes. Like blonde jokes, or ethnic jokes, or jabs that target husbands and wives or men and women in general, the fat joke is another subgenre of the put-down based on stereotyping and exaggeration.

Aside from residing in two eras -- one before and one after the digital revolution -- the two jokes above have one significant difference, and it has to do with whose big butt is the butt of the joke -- yours or mine. Clearly, saying "you" is insulting someone directly. The same joke with "I" or "me" changes everything.

The when and where of joke telling also has the power to bend the same words into different meanings. Before we as a nation increased our levels of empathy and tolerance (or just bit our lips in deference to political correctness), there was no escaping jokes that relied on hurtful stereotypes to attack large ethnic groups with a single punchine.

But time marches on, and people still like to laugh. Today, as minorities feel sufficiently empowered to make fun of themselves, Jewish, black and Latino comedians have resurrected ethnic humor for their kindred audiences and taken it to new extremes.

The edgy comics want you to think they are breaking the rules, but in two important ways, they're still playing it safe. They're making fun of themselves, and picking the right time and place to do it.

Fat jokes, I will argue, are equally permissible under the same limitations of appropriateness. We'll get to the rules, but first let's limber up the old funny bone with some victimless, food-based humor, beginning with the most reviled art form, the pun:

- Practice safe eating. Always use a condiment!

- Dijon vu is the same mustard as before!

- A hangover is the wrath of grapes!

- A boiled egg in the morning is hard to beat!

- Bakers share bread recipes on a knead-to-know basis!

Okay. Enough groaners. How about these?

- An optimist is a person who starts a diet on Thanksgiving Day!

- The First Law of Dietetics: If it tastes good, it's bad for you!

- If it weren't for coffee, I'd have no personality whatsoever!

- I don't even butter my bread. I consider that cooking!

- Life is uncertain. Eat dessert first!

- If animals were not meant to be eaten, why are they made of meat?

- Researchers have identified a food that diminishes the appetite for sex by 85 percent over two years. It's called a wedding cake!

- Women will never be the equal of men until they can hang out at a bar -- with a bald head and a beer gut -- and still think they're sexy!

- If you can't stick with the grapefruit diet, you're doing it wrong. Just eat everything but grapefruit!

- The government is considering a new nutritional labeling system. Foods will either be described as no fat, low fat, or fat but with a great personality!

- "There is no sincerer love than the love of food." ~ George Bernard Shaw.

- "How long does getting thin take?" ~ Winnie-the-Pooh.

- "Fishing is boring, unless you catch an actual fish. Then it's disgusting." ~ Dave Barry.

- "I Beat Anorexia!" ~ XXXL t-shirt.

A previous chapter dealt at length with the Fat Acceptance movement and its implications for you, society and the body politic. Suffice to say, fat pride starts at home, with you, your friends, and your family. It means loving yourself, calling a truce in the weight wars and cutting yourself some slack. Sometimes laughter is the best medicine. Really.

Laughing is good for you because it's hard on stress. With the first guffaw, oxygen flow increases, your heart, lungs and muscles lap it up, good-time endorphins begin to flow, and stress melts away. And that's just the immediate benefit. With regular doses of humor, your body can produce more of its natural painkillers and strengthen your immune system. Laughing makes it easier to connect with other people. It takes the edge off difficult situations and makes it easier to swallow life's bitter medicines.

Practice laughing at yourself and what others have to say, even when it's not funny. Then become a contributor to the laugh factory. But practice at home before treating your next Bible study or office meeting like an open mic night at the comedy club. Start with safe jokes and anecdotes. Can't remember a joke? Tell it three times in the mirror and it's yours for life. Build your repertoire until there is enough in your mental file cabinet to pull out just the right one for the right audience at the right time. When in doubt, keep your mouth shut. Then laugh at life. Try some bonding humor, the kind that says to your friends and co-workers "We're all in this together." And after you're comfortable with all of that, and your friends are laughing with you, and not out of pity, you might find just the right time to unveil a just-right, plump and juicy fat joke.

BUTTERFAT FUNNY

The lowly fat joke is not a new category we can blame on Comedy Central. In William Shakespeare's *Henry IV, Part 1*, one character is described as being "as fat as butter." Mae West, the full-figured comedienne who titillated Broadway and movie-goers in the 1930s, was happy to poke fun at her own, ample self. "I didn't discover curves; I only uncovered them," she come-hithered. "I never worry about diets," West said. "The only carrots that interest me are the number you get in a diamond." The platinum blonde fought regularly with censors and championed her belief that "those who are easily shocked should be shocked more often."

In the 1960s, the plus-sized comedienne Totie Fields spoke for a growing number of Americans when she said: "I've been on a diet for two weeks and all I've lost is two weeks." In the golden era of Saturday Night Live, John Belushi, John Candy and Chris Farley reasserted that nothing, including their own weight, was off-limits in the hunt for laughs, even if it killed them, and it sorta did. Today, regrettably, the fat joke category has been dominated by purveyors of the put-down. As a comedy cousin to rap music, the hip-hop movement has spawned hundreds of jokes beginning with the same four words: "Yo Mama so fat. . . "

For our purposes, the best thing to be said about "Yo Mama" jokes is that they can all can become less insulting but funnier just by switching the first two words to "I am." May I demonstrate?

- I am so fat, when I go to Golden Corral, I get a group discount.

- I am so fat, my cereal bowl came with a lifeguard.

- I am so fat, the last time I jumped up, I got stuck in mid-air.

- I was such a fat kid that when I ran away, they had to use all four sides of the milk carton.

Caution: It matters from where, in the heart, the joke is coming. Coupled with confidence, being the butt of a joke is brave. Self-described "losers" can make matters worse with the same put-down. There was even a large, blind study that showed the impact of an individual's status on how a joke is perceived.[309]

Here's an example, minus the fat factor. Whether he's giving a speech about the internet, energy policy or global warming, a Tennessean who is well qualified in all three areas likes to begin his remarks this way: "Hello. My name is Al Gore and I used to be the next president of the United States."

Bam! Gore's audience knows immediately that he is cool, confident, and smart enough not to take himself too seriously. The ice has been broken by the elephant in the room. Everything that follows the joke comes across as less threatening, more involving, more human.

Politicians, comedians and just-plain-Janes and Joes can all find opportunities to use self-deprecating humor as a way to become more approachable, both personally and professionally. Properly and judiciously executed, the occasional joke-on-me can break down barriers and open doors to communication.

Don't worry. Just by reading this book, you have pole position for a winning team. And if a joke flops, so what? It's a wisecrack, not a *NO REGERTS* neck tattoo.

ENCORE! ENCORE!

- I'm so fat, when a wear a red T-shirt, the kids expect Kool-Aid.

- I'm so fat, when I step on the scales, it says "Limit One Person."

- I'm so fat, I sat on a rainbow and made Skittles.

- I'm so fat, I can't even jump to conclusions.

- I'm so fat, I sat on a Wal-Mart and lowered the prices.

- I'm so fat, I can go on vacation just by rolling over.

- I'm so fat, I can step on a dollar bill and make change.

- I'm so fat, when I wore a yellow raincoat, someone yelled: "Taxi!"

309: Geoffrey F. Miller. "Dissing Oneself Versus Dissing Rivals: Effects of Status, Personality, and Sex on the Short-Term and Long-Term Attractiveness of Self-Deprecating and Other-Deprecating Humor." Evolutionary Psychology. 2008. Volume 6(3). Yep, there is a study about that.

- I'm so fat, when my pager beeps, people assume I'm backing up.

- I'm so fat, when I go into a restaurant, I just look at the menu and say, "Okay."

- I'm so fat, I had to go to Seaworld for my baptism.

- I'm so fat, when I go to the beach, the tide comes in.

- I'm so fat, when I rest on the beach, Greenpeace pushes me back in.

- I'm so fat, my senior pictures had to be an aerial view.

- I'm so fat, I'm on both sides of the family.

- I'm so fat, even my clothes have stretch marks.

- I'm so fat, small objects orbit around me.

- I'm so fat, my favorite food is seconds.

- I'm so fat, I'm once, twice, three times a lady.

- I'm so fat, my passport photo says, "Continued overleaf."

- I'm so fat, I deejay for the ice cream truck.

- I'm so fat, when the doctor diagnosed me with the flesh-eating disease, he gave me 12 years to live.

- I'm so fat, my blood type is alfredo.

- I'm so fat, when I get really hot, I smell like bacon.

- I'm so fat, I stay on a light diet. As soon as it's light, I start eating.

- I'm so fat, I'm half white, half black and half Hispanic.

- I'm so fat, I just need to gain five pounds to get group insurance.

- I'm so fat, when I stepped on a talking scale, it said: "Please step out of the car."

- I'm so fat, when I turn around my friends throw me a welcome back party.

- I'm so fat, my friends have to take a train, a bus and an Uber to get on my good side.

- I'm so fat, when my family wants to watch a home movie, they ask me to wear white.

- I'm so fat, my bathtub has stretch marks.

- I'm so fat, when I fell down, I rocked myself to sleep trying to get up.

- I'm so fat, ever since I stepped on our cat's tail, we've been calling him Beaver.

I hope you enjoyed these carefully chosen fat jokes. If not, please address your highly valued comments to: maewest@cypresshillscemetery.com.

25

LOOKY YOU!

ere's something to remember during an afternoon of poking through your closets and drawers to admire the pretty clothes that fit "the real you." The real you does not fit those clothes anymore.

Perhaps you are one of the few humans who truly have a widely fluctuating weight range. Fine. Keep it all. But if it's been a few years since the thin end of the rack got any use, accept the fact that almost everyone gradually thickens over the years. The unselfish thing to do is to give those clothes to someone who can wear them. Take them to Goodwill or a consignment shop and treat yourself to something stylish and new, something that fits and flatters.

Self-acceptance does wonders for the space between your ears. Using that same confidence to dress in a way that accentuates the positive and camouflages the rest will help everyone else notice the real you as a real person, not a blob of ambulating fat cells. All of us have seen heavy people who dress as if their only goal is to keep others a good 20 feet away. Fat acceptance doesn't mean confronting others with a take-it-or-leave-it disregard for your appearance. It means dressing and grooming in a way that communicates intelligence, comfortable confidence, and friendliness. And if a subtle makeover gradually leads to stronger friendships, blooming romance, or a big job promotion... well, you will just have to adjust to your new status.[310]

310: Your author doesn't mind some occasional uptown hours in a suit and tie, but normally dresses as if he only buys clothes during an annual visit to Myrtle Beach. And that would be true. For this chapter, I leaned heavily on my wife's keen sense of style, along with guidance from some ardcover volumes already in one of her many baskets of books. I acknowledge and honestly recommend these volumes:

MEN AND OTHER PROBLEM AREAS

I've been married long enough to know nothing is simple for women confronting their wardrobes, so let's quickly address the comparatively straightforward task of menswear and menswear-not.

Large men may unfairly have the advantage of projecting strength and authority. The important thing is to avoid projecting ridiculousness.

Nothing makes a man look fatter than having a belt positioned around the largest part of his equator. Pulling the pants up even higher only draws more attention to the lower abdomen, especially if the britches are stretched tight in the crotch to achieve the higher waist. Just ask the ladies how sexy that is. You may see the finger-to-open mouth gesture, a universal sign for gagging.

Men can soften the equator effect with a shirt and pants that are as stylish as a GQ model would wear, albeit large enough to fit loosely in any position. A loose-hanging jacket also helps to replace width with height.

Casual wear should take advantage of looser styles, minus the low-rider waists that tell us more than we want to know about a preference for boxers or briefs. Lean toward solid, muted colors. Save the loud prints for bowling, beaches and hailing rescue helicopters. The well-dressed executive need only follow the general rules of office decorum, being especially careful not to knot the necktie too short in an ill-advised nod to Dilbert. A spare tie in the desk drawer is an excellent investment. Nothing says "fat slob" like a cravat caked with lunch drippings. A tall, stovepipe hat will certainly emphasize height, but expect unwanted comparisons to Lincoln or Slash. So go with something more modest.

WOMEN WHO WEAR

Ladies, I know you think shoes make a huge difference in your total presentation, but unless you're wearing pink Chuck Taylors at the time of your abduction, most men will have no useful information to give the investigating

Leah Feldon. *Does This Make Me Look Fat? The Definitive Rules for Dressing Thin for Every Height, Size, and Shape.* Villard. New York. 2000.
Linda Dano with Anne Kyle. *Looking Great . . .Fashion Authority and Television Star Linda Dano Shares Her Style and Beauty Secrets To Help You Look Your Best.* G.P. Putnam's Sons. New York. 1997.
Charla Krupp. *How Not To Look Old: Fast and Effortless Ways to Look 10 Years Younger, 10 Pounds Lighter, 10 Times Better.* Springboard Press. New York. 2008.

officer. Obviously, heels add height. I'd say wear whatever you and your friends appreciate so long as you don't look like a medicine ball on stilts.

For casual wear, women who prefer to be understated at times should choose loose-fitting pants and a top in muted tones. Calm colors in a fitted waist or long vest will up the chic factor. When fun and flirting are on the agenda, there is no reason to avoid brighter colors and prints, so long as they are size-appropriate.

You'd think all this was common sense until you stroll through Sprawl-Mart on a Friday night. Bite your tongue while beholding the parade of bulging bare bellies, tattoos creeping out of gym shorts, and sweatpants stretched tight enough to turn ankles blue. Bad taste, like insect larvae, will always be with us. We pray for the day each chubby caterpillar will become a beautiful butterfly. For now, we quietly reflect on how all of us can use a little help.

Until recently, major clothing stores have hated on the heftier half. Any self-conscious teen who could be persuaded to go clothes shopping with thin friends knew what to expect: long aisles stocked with the latest fashions in a narrow range of small sizes. And in a distant corner, a single rack of "plus" size clothing dripped with shapeless shifts and dress prints that went out of style with 8-track tapes.

Large adult women with money to spend on something other than a pink muumuu have been equally frustrated, not only by the dearth of selection, but a reasonable suspicion they are not welcome in trendier stores. Shopping at fat-friendly stores such as Lane Bryant, Marina Rinaldi, Torrid and Hot Topic greatly expands the style options, but still smacks of apartheid for women and teens still struggling to love their fluffy selves. Shopping online affords adequate privacy, but eliminates the practical fun of trying on different styles and sizes in a trendy fashion outlet pumped up with lighting, music, fragrance, and your own cheering section.

Good news! After an earlier attempt short-circuited by the recession, mainstream clothing retailers are again giving plus sizes some respect. This is no doubt because (Choose one):

1. The clothing industry is feeling much remorse about its disdainful treatment of heavy women for a hundred years and wants to make things right, or

2. After clinging to the idea that 14 and 16 are plus sizes -- even though it's now the average size for American women -- losses sustained in the downturn have forced marketers to embrace a big, fat fact: Sales of "plus-sized" clothing are close to $20 billion per year but could be doubled if retailers really went after the market segment's actual buying power.

One survey that is already outdated showed that 40 percent of women wear plus sizes, compared to only 30 percent each for regular and junior sizes.

Perhaps Apple and Facebook can afford to leave that kind of money on the table, but not clothiers. Their labor and production costs are high, and getting a little higher with the extra fabric required to drape real women.

Now, even the makers of wedding gowns are sheepishly participating in full-figured fashion shows while trying not to offend the idealized customers long targeted for brand identification. Department stores are adding larger sizes of the same styles offered to middleweights. And heavier models, at least by fashion industry standards, are showing up in catalogs unheralded and unnoticed, simply because they, too, can look great in the right outfits.

There is so much potential for the fashion industry to build goodwill and revenue by respecting a *Fat, Smart and Happy* population. It may take a few more years for designers to accept that 180-pound women come in a variety of shapes, but retailers that get there first with the best range of fits will be making friends for life.

FIT, FABRIC AND FLUSTER

Size matters. It would be nice if sizing mattered too. For the most part, we're stuck with an off-the-rack sizing system that defies logic and consistency. Grrrr, huh? So stick with with two or three stores and three or four brands that usually fit you. Let the dressing room mirrors help you adjust the color level, tints and contrast.

Because I am neither a professional fat person nor an amateur crossdresser, I have weighed advice about achieving full-figured style from multiple female sources and filtered it with my own heterosexual dude logic. You should disagree with me often. We're not designing a fat uniform. Style is, above all, personal.

"Slimming" can be overrated. Look for styles which will flatter your curves in the right place at the right time. Men are easily impressed by an ample bosom, according to my wife's husband. This doesn't mean you want to look like a top-heavy pole dancer. With great cleavage comes great responsibility. Even Hollywood starlets save their best décolletage for the red carpet or a brief movie scene (which the guys in the marketing department will certainly include in the preview trailer and ads on TV).

For most situations, a dark top with a large round neck or shallow V-neck will draw only the right amount of inspection. Avoid lapel pins and necklaces which draw attention too far below that pretty face. Save the strapless dresses for evening wear and soft lighting, or perhaps casual Fridays at the office if the air conditioning is failing. A $20 personal fan for your desk is also a great investment.

There's nothing intrinsically right or wrong about wearing a dress, assuming your daily routine is free of cartwheels and somersaults. Prints require extra consideration to shape and color, but a nice fit with eye appeal beats a shapeless black tent any day. Vertical patterns can accentuate height while an empire waist magically enhances a disproportionately small bosom and diverts attention from plump hips. A versatile wrap or shawl affords flexible fit from the neck to the knees any time of the day or month. Ignore how a dress looks on a model. That's just bait and switch. Pay attention to how the dress's collar, sleeves, color and cut look on *you*.

Select fabrics and sizes that drape a little. Spandex isn't magic. The greater its tug, the more bulges are highlighted. If it hurts, it's too tight.

Regarding short tops over bare bellies: Don't. Just don't. Avoid pants with a low-rise waist unless your top is long enough to cover the rest. Choose tops with subtle vertical ribs or stripes. Horizontal stripes can work if worn with a jacket to break up the widescreen presentation.

Sleeveless tops are generally counter-productive. If you're proud of your flabby arms, good for you. But most of the people you encounter will judge you by the untamed wiggling and pay less attention to your words of wisdom. A light jacket with flowing sleeves and waist converts that bulk to beauty.

Always wear baggy T-shirts -- if you want to look like a big person in a baggy T-shirt. But why would you? Choose tees with a gentle fit, not a tight one.

Pants with stirrups: Not ever. Light athletic wear is equally comfortable and far more flattering, assuming there is sufficient room for the hips and legs. Men can be stupid, but very few are interested in trying to bounce a dime off your butt.

For work and other public appearances, choose pants with straight lines and a straight cut. A snug fit at the ankles only enlarges the appearance of everything above. Don't go baggy; that's just as bad. Avoid pleats, oversized pockets and prominent zippers. If you can't find a shape that fits and flatters, spend a little on the tailoring needed to get it just right. Your butt will thank you, as will all those who follow in your footsteps.

Female professionals need suits to accentuate their position and poise. Quality matters, but what looks great on the rack or in a catalog will come off as a cheap burlesque if the size and fit aren't right. Longer, single-breasted jackets will always trump short, boxy designs. A little tapering around the waist works if the bust and hips contribute to an hourglass effect. Sophisticated variations in a comfortable blouse, scarf, jewelry and handbag extend the appeal and variety of suits worn in heavy rotation. Traveling or not, you always want to look like you're flying first-class, not in a dog crate.

Office and retail workers who punch a time clock aren't excused from dressing for success. Things to leave at home: sweatpants, frayed jeans, mini skirts, low-cut or see-through tops, worn-out tennis shoes, and strapless tops without a jacket. Classy and comfortable can be the same thing, from hair accessories to shoes. Take your cues from your best-dressed colleagues, not the worst. Yes, these rules should apply to female co-workers of every size. No, they are not measured and enforced uniformly. Whether deliberately of unconsciously, your supervisor is making mental notes that may affect your evaluation for pay and promotion. So play along. It's like earning a new and better wardrobe.

Save your loudest, most comfortable clothing for exercise and other activities. Start with a proper-fitting sports bra so that you know where your breasts are at all times.

Swimwear: Here's one occasion when a mini-skirt does a body good. Fashion be damned, swimsuits with legs cut high to the waist only provide a showcase for saddlebags and thunder thighs. String bikinis should never leave the backyard. Enjoy the surf and sun with a nice one-piece that promotes freckles on top of the bosom and shade below. Dark, matte colors are usually the way to go, perhaps with colorful accents and a wide-brimmed hat to keep it interesting. Rules aside, whatever contributes to your confidence is worth a try. Shopping for swimwear should, at the least, be more fun than a Pap smear. Take a trusted friend to share some honest opinions as you try on several candidates. Once you've settled on some works of art and put them on public display, keep the colors and elastic fresh by rinsing out the chlorine, salt water or perspiration in fresh water after each outing.

No matter what the occasion, the one question honest men prefer not to answer is "Does this make me look fat?" To keep the peace, I suggest that my lady try on two or three options, so she can ask me which one I like best.

"Gosh, Honey," I'll say. "You decide. They all look great!"

Because I wasn't born Monday.

FIRST IMPRESSIONS

If you dress to make a fool of yourself or to keep strangers at a distance, then you're well-positioned for a life of loneliness and self-loathing. But even if you smartly choose to dress to impress, remember that clothes don't do all the talking. Walk with a relaxed, approachable confidence. A friendly smile, positive body language and a genuine interest in others will make a huge difference, whether you're in the company of strangers, co-workers or old friends. Even if your habits and instincts seem to be serving you well, pay attention to basic skills and trying to see yourself as others see the real you -- not just your clothes -- and you will always find room for improvement. The basics:

Smile when you meet someone. No, it's not cool to appear thoughtful and aloof. Ditch the disinterested air. Opt for inviting, affirming and likeable. Many ladies of the South instinctively embrace this charm offensive and increase it, when appropriate, by another 11 to 37 percent -- sort of like writers who make up such numbers to inflate their grasp of the facts.

A firm -- not painful -- handshake is always appropriate, especially for women. Eye contact, vigor and duration (measured in milliseconds) all contribute to instantly telegraphing your confidence and assertiveness. Okay, that's long enough. Let go and let your smile do the talking.

Stay in the moment with those around you. Talk about what's happening right now, unless, perchance, you awoke this morning with your head in a bear's mouth. That always makes a good story. Otherwise, avoid one-upmanship. If you catch yourself saying: "If you think that's something," finish with: "Well, you're right!"

Introduce yourself where appropriate and invite others to join in your conversation.

Ask questions. If you don't like the way the chit-chat is going, use a different question to gently switch tracks on the conversation. If somehow the topic moves to dieting and weight, listen long enough the gauge the direction it's headed, then contribute as much as you want with just the right amount of wisdom, empathy, rebuttal and humor. Regard weight as a popular topic, like the weather, politics or Hollywood gossip, not as a touchy subject or as measure of anyone's health, character, or personality.

Then love yourself more for reacting like an expert without acting like a know-it-all. And darned if you didn't look good doing it!

FINAL WORDS
(WAFER THIN)

It's a big, fat, crowded planet. But you're the only you.

All the wisdom and advice in the world cannot take you where you don't want to go. Be grateful for that. Personal freedom means accepting responsibility for bad judgment and enjoying the rewards of smart decisions. The challenging part, as it relates to weight and health, is that the result of good choices made today can take weeks, months, even years, to manifest. No biggie. You can stay busy living your life, free from blame, free from guilt and free to be whoever you want.

Again, talk to friends, family and medical professionals before making any big changes. You will want their support later. But if you never lose a pound or eat another carrot or park a little further away from the door, and even if you simply reject all the science and opinions in these pages, please indulge this one request:

Don't let body weight influence the respect you have for yourself and others. It is lazy and hurtful to consider body fat a measure of anyone's character. After spending all this time together, I happen to know you're much better than that. And I'm pretty sure that right now, or in a time and place of your choosing, you deserve some quality chocolate.

I absolutely loved our time together.
Thank you so much for having me over.

Ciao! (I'll just quietly let myself out.)